Classiq Cooking

21

Meals and Drinks
to Satisfy your Classiq Palate

Dawn Classiq

Classiq Cooking

21

Meals and Drinks
to Satisfy your Classiq Palate

Cooking is a way to bring people together to enjoy happy meals. Food makes people happy. Each bite, each mistake, each taste and feeling that food gives you is incomparable. So why write a cookbook? To cultivate, inspire and engage people through food, workouts and drinks. It's my way of sharing my newly found knowledge, motivation and a way to give back! So, I hope you are inspired and enjoy this small token of my appreciation.

To my "greatest achievement:" Thank you for ALWAYS believing in me and continuing to push and motivate me when I was lost.

———————

To my mom: Thank you for your endless support and having the desire to be a part of my many adventures. Even when they don't make sense.

———————

To my food artist: Eat. Workout. Drink. REPEAT!!!

———————

To the queen that lives within me: Thank you for never giving up on yourself. Who knew that your darkest moments would birth something so beautiful? Praise God!

XO ~ Dawn Classiq

I dedicate this book to my grandmother,
Bernice Landon.
Grandma, thanks for inspiring me! I love you
and know that you are smiling and guiding
my footsteps.

Your chocolate drop

To my fellow food artist,

Please keep in mind that you can't have a dish without disclaimers. Below are a few imperative notes that you'll need to know before reading any further. I truly believe that I owe you, my joyful food artist, the utmost care and diligence before using this cookbook as a guide or reference to maintaining a healthy lifestyle. Please read the disclaimers entirely before beginning.

Medical disclaimer:

1. The information provided in this book is for educational purposes only, and does not substitute for professional medical advice.

2. Consult a medical professional or healthcare provider if you're seeking medical advice, diagnoses, or treatment.

No responsibility Disclaimer:

1. Although the publisher and the author have made every effort to ensure that the information in this book was correct at press time and while this publication is designed to provide accurate information in regard to the subject matter covered, the publisher and the author assume no responsibility for errors, inaccuracies, omissions, or any other inconsistencies herein and hereby disclaim any liability to any party for any loss, damage, or disruption caused by errors or omissions, whether such errors or omissions result from negligence, accident, or any other cause.

2. This publication is meant as a source of valuable information for the reader, however it is not meant as a substitute for direct expert assistance. If such level of assistance is required, the services of a competent professional should be sought.

Views expressed Disclaimer:

1. The views and opinions expressed here are those of the author and do not necessarily reflect the official policy or position of other licensed professionals. Any content provided by the author is of their opinion and not intended to malign any religion, ethnic group, club, organization, company nor individual.

Investment Disclaimer:

1. The author takes no responsibility on how others act based on the advice given in this book.

2. DO YOUR OWN RESEARCH: The content is intended to be used and must be used for informational purposes only. It is very important to do your own research before making any health related decisions based on your own personal circumstances. You should take independent advice from a health professional, in connection with, or independently research and verify any information that you find in this book and wish to rely upon for all purposes.

CONTENTS

Classiq Cooking

21

Meals and Drinks
to Satisfy your Classiq Palate

A guide to enhance and enrich lives through healthy food options, at-home fitness, and delicious drinks bursting with flavor!

> » Before preparing each meal, be sure to rinse all vegetables, fruits, and seafood thoroughly prior to cooking.

> » Gluten Free will be referred to as GF in all recipes that call for it.

> » Vegetarian will be referred to as VG in all recipes that call for it.

INTRODUCTION

Staying in shape is arguably one of the most challenging life tasks there is. We all work so hard to look our best 100% of the time. "Eat healthy", "workout everyday", use tools such as fad diets, waist trainers and surgery to have a "perfect body" and "enhance our beauty." Society tells us all these same lame beliefs. Truth is, nothing or no one will be perfect 100% of the time. However, we can find peace in striving to be the best version of ourselves, IF we dedicate ourselves to do the work, daily.

This book couldn't have come at a better time in my life. Mentally, I was experiencing significant changes in my life, and despite all my accolades and life successes, I felt stifled and complacent. Working on this book helped me work through all that I was feeling. You see, cooking has always been a part of my upbringing and continues to help guide, build and nurture relationships. I've also known that it is necessary to implement a balanced workout to go along with balanced meals. Classiq Cooking shares techniques and tips on how to do that.

It took me a while to truly live by this practice, but once I started balancing my life with the things that truly make me feel good and gifting my body with healthy attention, I started discovering my best self. This practice has made me realize why it is so important that we strive each day to be the best version of ourselves and to create a guilt-free atmosphere while doing it. So lastly, I dedicate this book to you; the person who struggles every day to be a better version of themselves than they were yesterday.

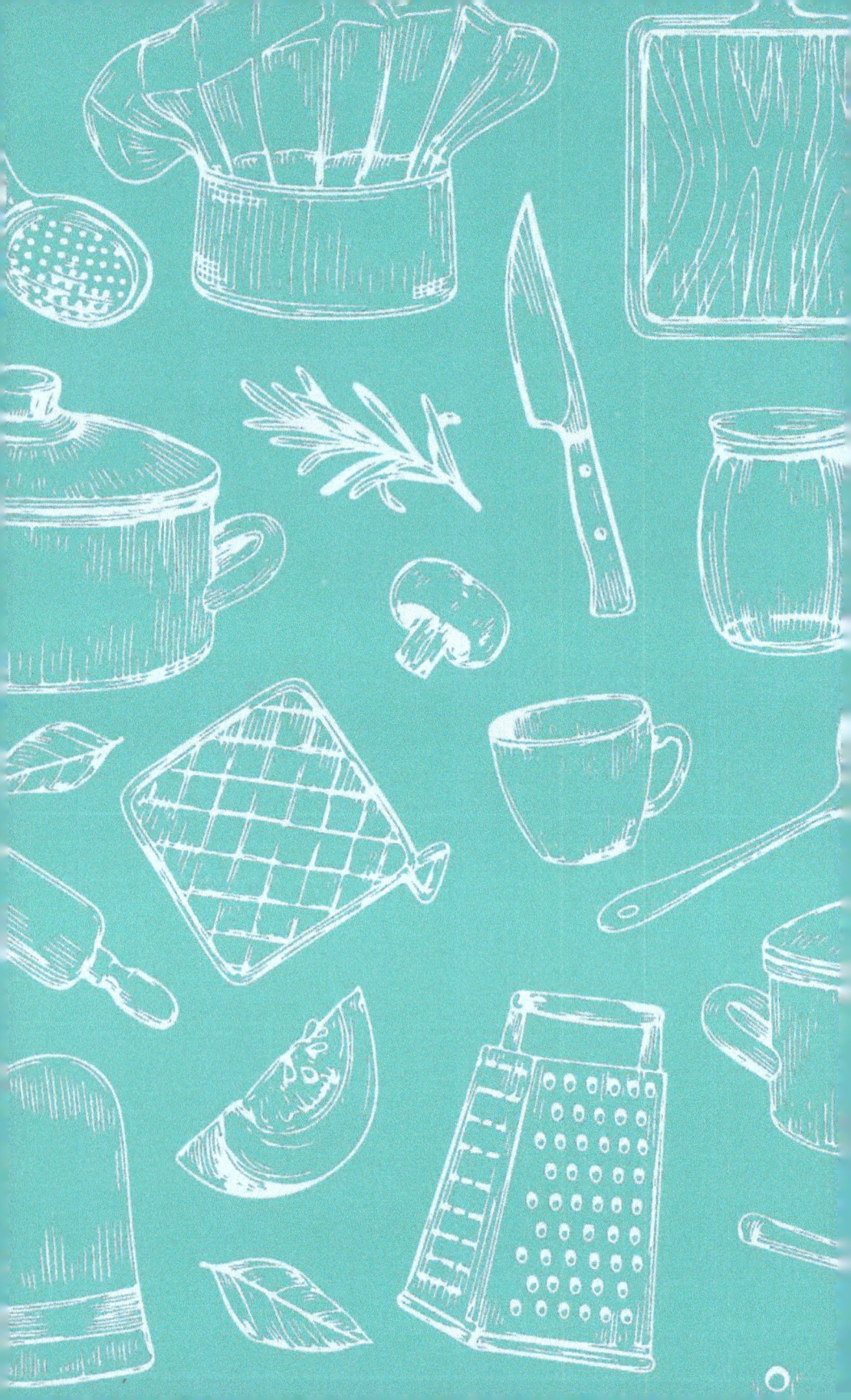

Classiq

COOKING

THE
SUNRISE
SELECTION

THE GOURMET BREAKFAST SANDWICH (VG)

Hmm, don't you just love a warm, flaky and cheesy breakfast sandwich? I know I do! This sandwich is perfect to impress any crowd and easy to make. Follow these steps below and create your morning masterpiece.

- 1 plant based breakfast sausage meat patty (I use Gardein)
- 1 egg
- 1 slice American cheese
- halved croissant
- 1 tbsp grape jelly
- 1 tsp salt
- 1 tsp black pepper
- 1 tbsp Mexican blend shredded cheese
- ½ tbsp butter
- 1 tbsp almond milk
- 1 tbsp olive oil (or oil of your preference)

SERVES
1

Preheat oven to 325°F

Lightly oil your baking sheet with olive oil. Slice the croissant in half and spread a thin layer of butter on the inside of both halves. Once the oven has reached 325°F, place the croissant halves on the baking sheet and insert in the oven on the middle rack for 5-8 minutes.

While the croissant halves are toasting, lightly coat the surface of a small non-stick skillet and place over low-medium heat. Add the patty and occasionally flip it. Cook for 8 minutes. Once the patty is cooked, slice the sausage in half and layer it on the bottom half of the croissant.

Combine the egg, butter, Mexican shredded cheese, salt, black pepper and almond milk in a large mixing bowl and whisk ingredients together.

Place your non-stick skillet over medium heat and pour in your eggs. Use a spatula to slowly push the eggs from one side to the other, making sure all the uncooked eggs touch the skillet. The eggs are finished once all loose contents are cooked and appear fluffy.

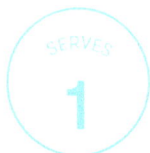

Next, layer your eggs directly on top of the sausage. Lastly, take your sliced cheese and layer it on top of your eggs. Allow the sandwich to continue warming in the oven for at least 1-2 minutes.

Take the sandwich out of the oven and top with grape jelly as desired. Close your sandwich with the top half of the croissant and enjoy!

Classiq Tip:

You can top your sandwich off with any desired Jelly or Jam. The most important tip is to not overcook the veggie patty. They cook faster than blinking twice.

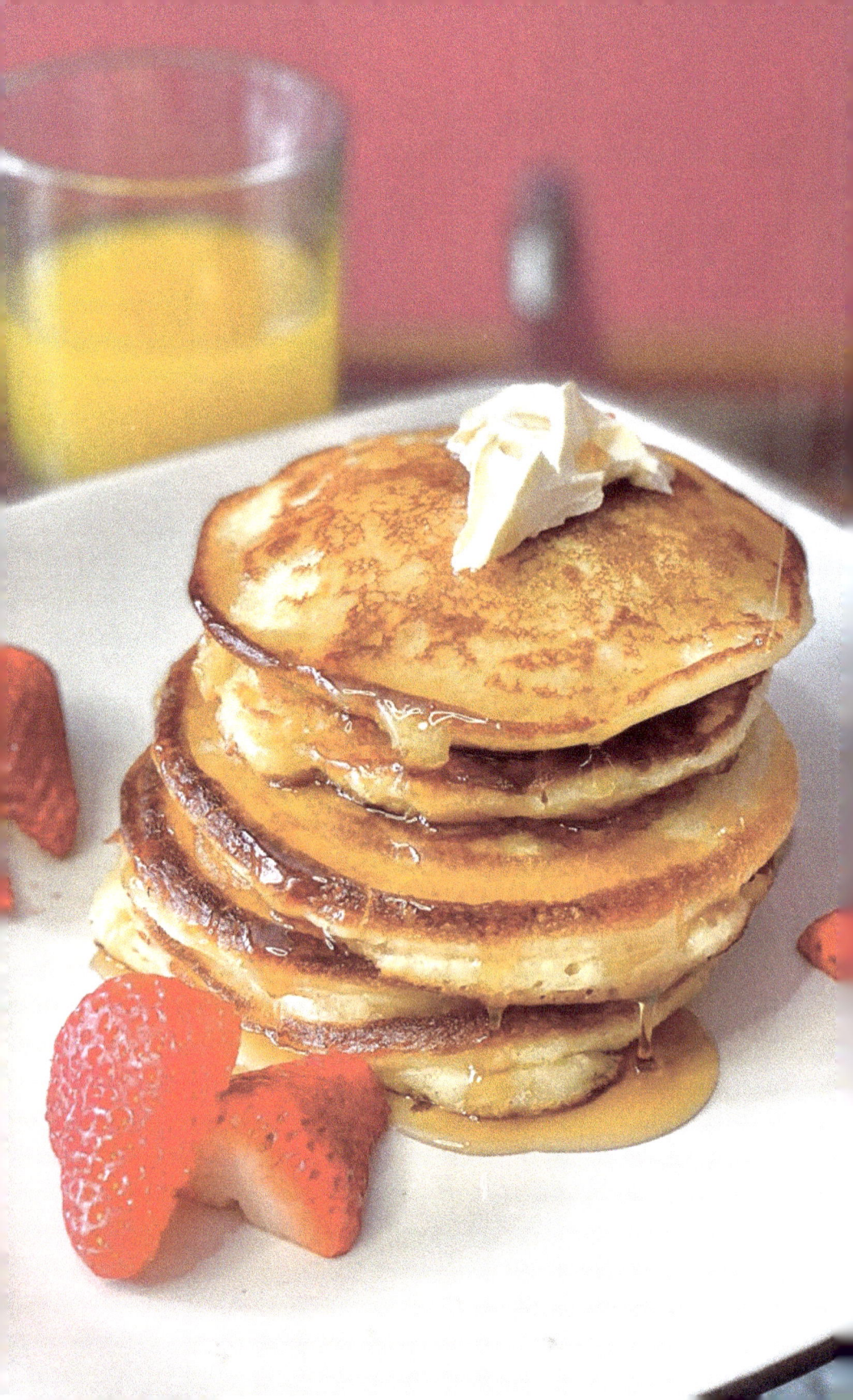

FLUFFY GLUTEN-FREE PANCAKES ⓥⓖ

Many people believe that Gluten-Free dishes aren't worth the time, but trust me when I say that this pancake recipe is unmatched! Get ready to experience a pancake like no other. If you love a good fluffy pancake with crispy and brown edges, don't wait to make this breakfast baddie. I can just taste it right now, melting in my mouth like butter. So what are you waiting for?...

- 1 cup all purpose GF flour (I use Pillsbury)
- 1 tsp pure vanilla extract
- 1 large egg
- 1 tbsp GF baking powder
- ¼ tsp salt
- ¾ cup almond milk
- 2 tbsp granulated sugar
- 3 tbsp olive oil (or oil of your preference)

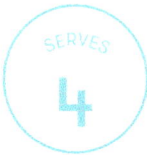

SERVES

4

Pour flour mix, baking powder, sugar and vanilla extract in a bowl and mix. Whisk in egg and almond milk. After the mixture has a paste-like consistency, warm 1 tbsp of olive oil in a skillet over low to medium heat. Once the oil is hot, pour in the pancake mix making 3 ½" - 4" wide circles.

The pancake mix will start to puff and create a bubble-like pattern on the edge of the top layer. This is a sign that the bottom side is almost done and is ready to be flipped. Flip pancake onto its opposite side for 1-2 minutes. Once the pancakes are golden brown on each side and have a nice crispy edge, plate and then top with butter, syrup or your favorite topping and enjoy!

Classiq Tip:

Did you know Gluten is a group of seed storage proteins found in certain cereal grains and provides no essential nutrients? Millions of people are affected by eating gluten because of the harsh impact it has on their immune system or they just have a difficult time digesting it.

"

Whatever you fuel
your body with, will
ultimately fuel you.

DELIGHTFUL EGG WHITE VEGGIE OMELET (GF) (VG)

The best thing about an egg white omelet is that it leaves you feeling light and full, giving you the energy you'll need for the rest of your day. This is my go-to after an early morning workout.

- 4 large eggs (or ¾ cup of egg whites in carton)
- ¼ cup sliced mushrooms
- ¼ cup green bell peppers, sliced
- ½ cup spinach
- ⅓ cup cherry tomatoes, halved
- 1 tbsp Feta cheese (or cheese of your choice)
- 1 ½ tbsp Mexican blend shredded cheese
- 1 tsp salt
- 1 tsp black pepper
- 1 tsp onion powder
- 1 tsp garlic salt
- ½ tsp onion and herb seasoning
- 1 tbsp GF soy sauce
- 1 tbsp butter
- ⅛ cup almond milk
- 1 tbsp olive oil

Add egg whites, butter, Mexican shredded cheese and almond milk into a large mixing bowl and whisk together. Then add salt and black pepper to taste.

Add 1 tbsp of olive oil to the skillet and warm over low to medium heat. Add the sliced bell pepper, tomatoes and mushroom. As the vegetables saute, season with onion powder, garlic salt and onion and herb seasoning. Continue to stir the veggies while they are cooking.

After about 2-3 minutes add the spinach and season with soy sauce, onion powder and black pepper. Once the spinach has cooked down, remove from heat and set aside.

Pour egg whites in a non-stick skillet and cook over medium heat allowing the bottom of the omelet to cook. Spread the vegetables evenly on top of the egg. When the bottom of the egg whites are golden brown, flip or fold the omelet in half and cook for 2-3 more minutes. Remove from heat and top with feta cheese.

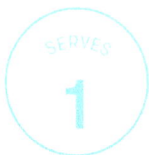

SERVES
1

Classiq Tip:

Egg whites are high in protein, but low in calories, fat and cholesterol!!!

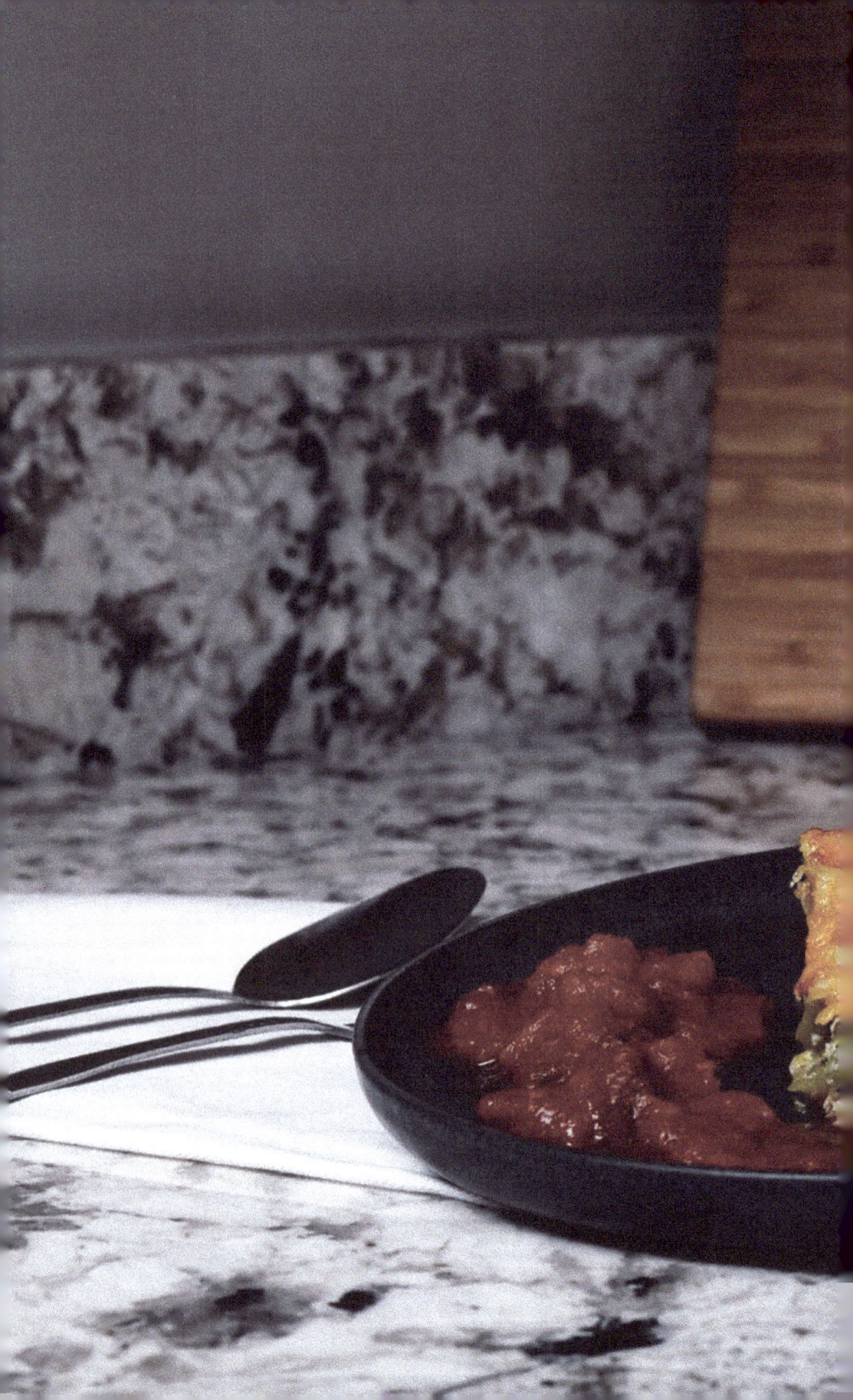

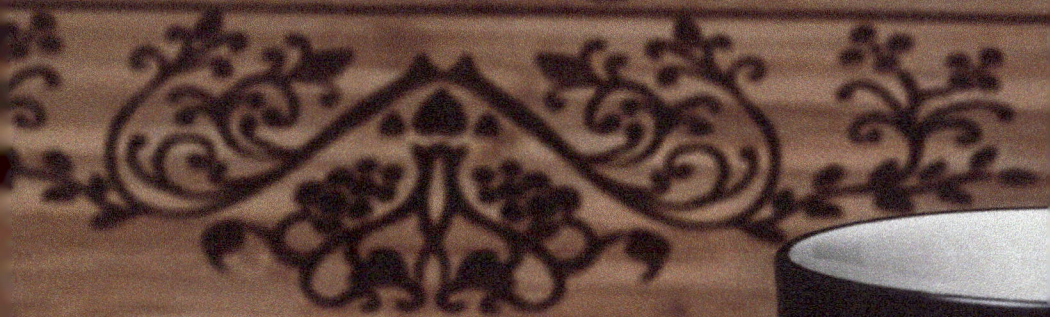

SCRUMPTIOUS VEGGIE EGG SOUFFLÉ (GF) (VG)

Yum, this dish is one of my favorite morning recipes. With so many veggies, this dish packs a nutritional balance that will leave you feeling completely satisfied. Eat it with a side of sour cream and salsa or eat it alone. Whatever you choose, I bet you'll come back for seconds.

- 7 eggs
- ½ green bell pepper and ½ red bell pepper, sliced
- 4 ozs fresh spinach
- 1 ½ cup fresh broccoli
- 1 cup mushrooms
- ½ cup onions
- 1 cup sharp cheddar shredded cheese
- 2 tbsp salt
- 2 tbsp black pepper
- 1 tsp seasoning salt
- 1 tbsp onion powder
- ½ tbsp garlic salt
- 1 tbsp onion and herb seasoning
- 1 tsp GF soy sauce
- 2 tbsp olive oil
- 5 tbsp butter
- ½ cup almond milk

Preheat the oven to 325 degrees. While the oven is warming, use a cutting board and cut off the broccoli stem and discard.

Add eggs, butter, cheese and almond milk into a large mixing bowl and whisk ingredients together. Then whisk in seasoning salt and black pepper.

Warm olive oil in a large skillet over low to medium heat then add in the broccoli, sliced bell peppers, onions and mushrooms. Saute the veggies while adding onion powder, garlic salt and onion and herb seasoning and continue to stir the vegetables with a spatula. After about 2-3 minutes, add spinach to the skillet. Season the spinach with GF soy sauce. Once the spinach has cooked down, pour the ingredients into the mixing bowl with the egg mixture.

Pour the egg-vegetable mixture into a non-stick pyrex pan and place on the middle rack of the oven. Bake for 15-20 minutes or until golden brown. While in the oven, top with cheese and allow the souffle to cool before plating.

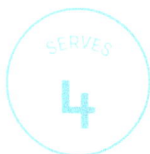

SERVES

4

Classiq Tip:

Whole eggs contain a variety of vitamins, minerals, extra protein and some healthy fats.

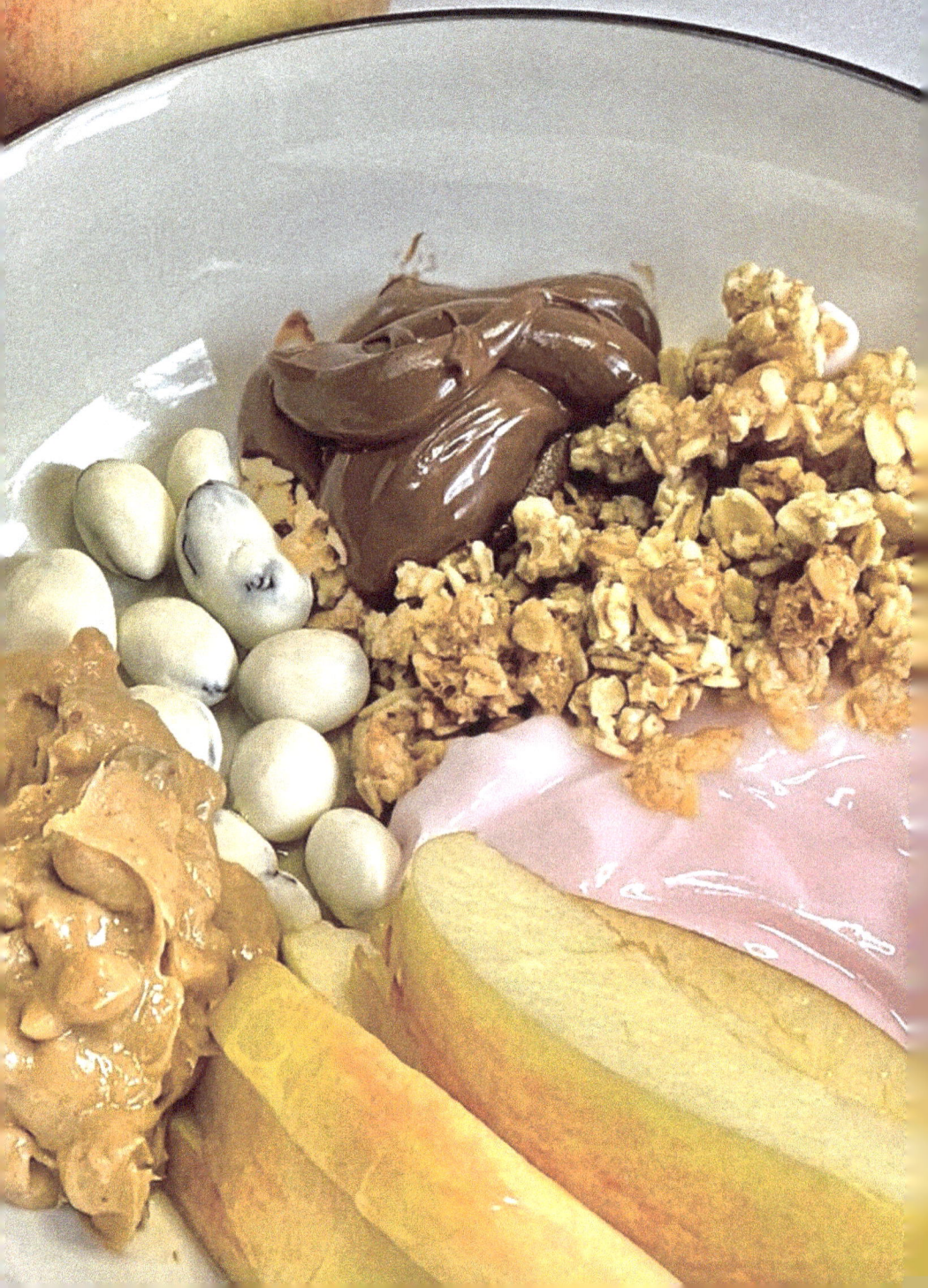

YUMMY PEANUT BUTTER BOWL (GF) (VG)

If you love peanut butter, you'll love this morning breakfast bowl. It's a great treat for both kids and adults. It's super easy to make and extremely yummy. Whether it's a weekday or the weekends, the PBB is set to fit your classiq palette. Dig into this recipe below:

- 3 tbsp peanut butter with peanut pieces
- ½ apple
- ¼ cup GF granola with raisins
- 6 ozs strawberry yogurt
- 1 tbsp honey
- 2 tbsp Nutella (can be substituted for any softened chocolate of your choice)

Layer the bottom of a bowl with half of the strawberry yogurt. Add half of the granola and layer it evenly along with the raisins on top of the yogurt. Cut the apple into thin slices and add an even layer on top of the granola. Drizzle honey over the top of the sliced apples. Add the other half of your yogurt on top of the apple followed by another layer of granola. Lastly, add a layer of peanut butter and a layer of Nutella.

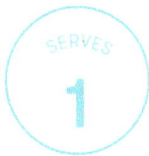

SERVES

1

Classiq Tip:

Peanut butter is a great source of protein. So turn this light breakfast into a fun snack for kids. Just ditch the bowl and yogurt and use sliced apples as your base!

CHEESY BREAKFAST POTATOES (GF) (VG)

Baby, these breakfast potatoes are sure to make you dance. It's like having a party in your mouth. Once the flavorful and soft potato reaches your tongue, you'll think it's sinfully delicious. This is definitely a crowd favorite. Look below to get the party started:

- 4 large potatoes, skin on
- 1 large onion
- ½ red bell pepper, ½ green bell pepper and ½ yellow bell pepper
- ½ cup Mexican blend shredded cheese
- 2 tsp onion powder
- 2 tsp garlic powder
- 2 tsp black pepper
- 2 tsp onion and herb seasoning
- 2 tsp garlic salt
- ½ cup olive oil

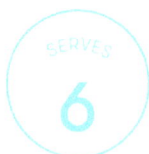

SERVES
6

Place potatoes in boiling water over high heat for 15-20 minutes or until potatoes are soft. Remove from heat, let cool on a cutting board, then slice into thin to medium thick slices. Season the potatoes with garlic salt, pepper, onion powder, garlic powder and onion and herb seasoning.

Slice onion and bell peppers and pour half of the oil in a large non-stick skillet and heat on low to medium. While the oil is warming add in the onion and bell peppers and saute them in the skillet with salt and black pepper for 5-8 minutes and then add in the seasoned potatoes. Pour the remaining oil over the top of the potatoes, occasionally adding a thin even layer of oil to ensure that the potatoes are lightly frying. Turn the heat up to medium and flip potatoes and veggies consistently for 10-15 minutes.

Top the potatoes off with cheese, cover them with a lid for 1-2 minutes. Allow the cheese to melt completely and serve.

Classiq Tip:

Boiling potatoes cuts down the cook time. I also use this technique for my fully loaded baked potatoes!

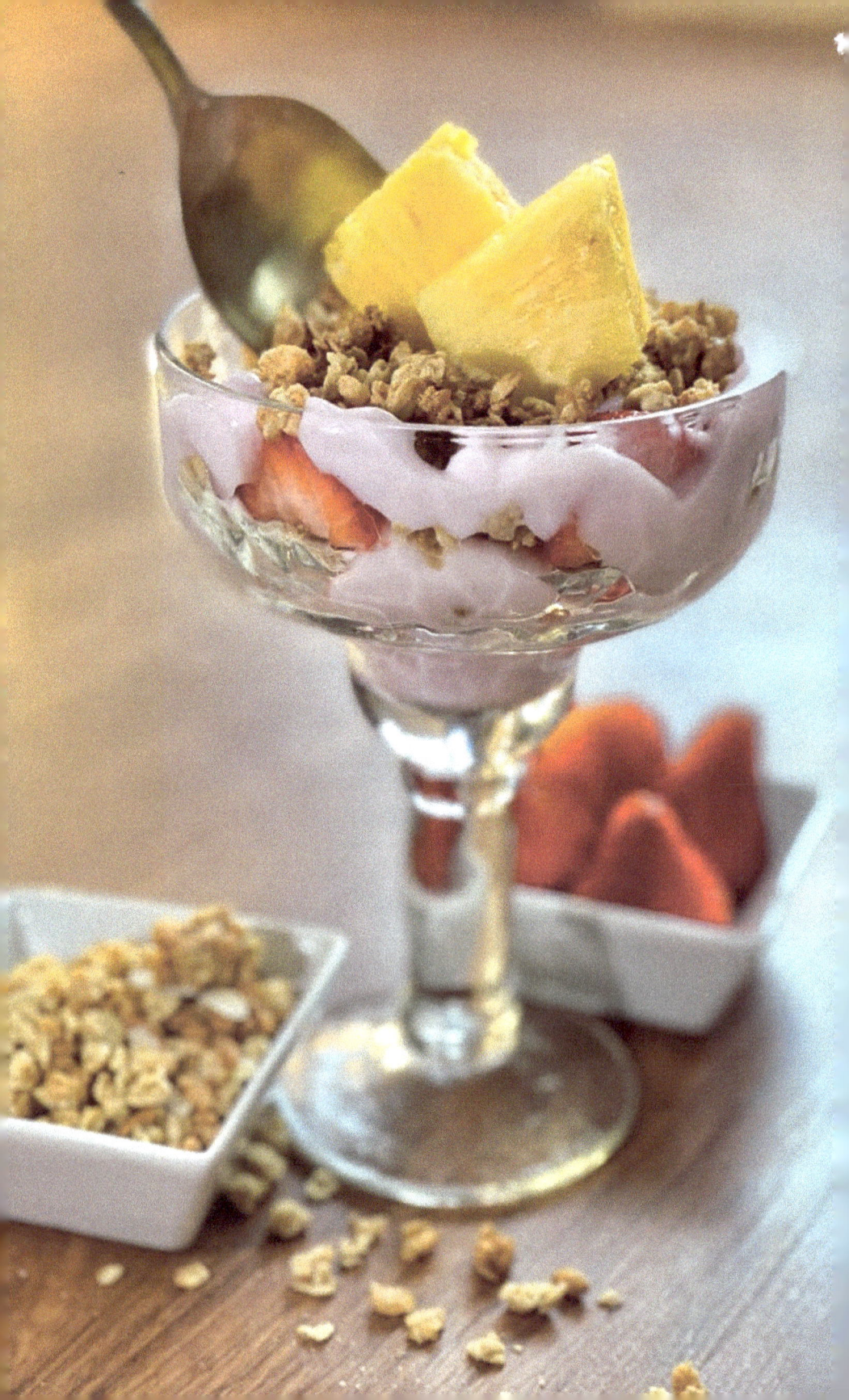

CLASSIQ CREAMY FRUIT & YOGURT PARFAIT (GF) (VG)

Who doesn't love a good parfait? It's like having dessert for breakfast and not feeling guilty. The best way to pair pineapples and strawberries is in our Classiq Parfait. This is the perfect way to start your dynamic day!

- 6 oz strawberry almond yogurt
- ¼ cup GF honey roasted granola
- 1 tsp honey
- 3 chunks pineapples
- 3 large strawberries

Spoon half of the yogurt into a glass first. Then layer half of the granola on top. Next, cut the calyx (leaf on the top of the strawberry) off, slice the strawberries into fours and pineapples into two. Then throw in half the strawberries and pineapples. Drizzle honey on top of the fruit. Repeat layering the ingredients and enjoy!

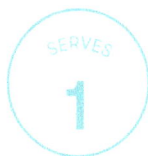

SERVES
1

Classiq Tip:

If you want to impress a crowd, use a champagne flute! Honestly, who doesn't love eating fruit out of an elegant glass while holding out their pinky?

CHAPTER

2

THE
MIDDAY
MUNCHIES

HONEY CRUSTED JERK SALMON ⓖⒻ

Anyone who's ever had a good piece of Salmon knows its juicy, yet flaky taste can be mouth-wateringly sinful. Hooonnneeeyyy, wait until you try my spin on it. It's delightful sweet and jerk taste is more than a gift, it's a blessing. Be careful because this recipe will surely have you overindulging. Now let's get started...

- 2 fresh salmon filets (skinless)
- 2 tbsp Jerk seasoning (check bonus recipe)
- 3 tbsp Honey Glaze Sauce (check bonus recipe)
- 1 tsp salt
- 1 tsp black pepper
- 1 tbsp olive oil
- 1 cup GF rosemary and olive oil multi-seed crackers (I use liveGfree brand)

Preheat oven to 425 degrees

Season the salmon on both sides with salt, pepper and Jerk seasoning. Next, in a small ziplock bag, crush the crackers and use them to coat both sides of your filet. Cover the bottom of the skillet with olive oil and lightly fry each side for 2-3 minutes on medium heat.

Grease the pyrex pan with a thin layer of olive oil and lay both filets flat side down. Bake in the oven for 5-8 minutes. This will allow the salmon to cook thoroughly. Before removing the salmon from the oven, drizzle the honey glaze directly on top and serve!

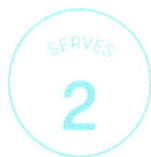

SERVES

2

Classiq Tip:

Did you know that salmon is a rich source of Omega-3 fatty acids and potassium? Salmon is also a powerhouse of proteins, vitamins and minerals. However, you shouldn't consume more than 2 servings per week due to the high levels of lead, mercury and other chemicals often ingested and stored in salmon.

THE VERY VEGGIE SUB (VG)

Get ready for a gooey, cheesy, flavor filled sandwich. You won't be able to deny how delightful this sandwich is. Once you take your first bite, you won't be able to stop. You'll soon realize that not all sandwiches need meat. Try this recipe and tell me what you think!

- 1 Italian Sub (I use Schwebel's brand)
- 3 medium mushrooms, sliced
- 1 cup green, red, yellow bell peppers, sliced
- 3 tbsp diced banana peppers
- ⅓ cup onion
- 1 tbsp GF soy sauce
- 3 tbsp olive oil
- ⅓ cup mozzarella cheese
- 1 tsp garlic salt
- 1 tsp roasted garlic and herb seasoning
- 1 tsp onion powder
- 1 tsp sea salt
- 1 tsp black pepper

Heat 2 tablespoons of oil in a large non-stick skillet and then saute onions, mushrooms, green, red, and yellow bell peppers for 8-10 minutes or until veggies have softened. While the vegetables are cooking, season them with soy sauce, garlic salt, pepper, sea salt, onion powder and garlic and herb seasoning. Next, place a lid on the top of the skillet and periodically stir the contents while the veggies simmer. As the veggies are finishing, top with banana peppers and mozzarella cheese and allow the cheese to melt.

Heat remaining oil on low to medium heat in a medium skillet and lightly toast the inner sides of the sub. Once the sub is golden brown, add the veggies onto one half of the sub, then your choice of condiments and finally cover with the other half of the sub. Enjoy!

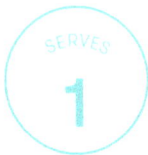

SERVES

1

Classiq Tip:

Don't overcook your veggies!!! While I hate undercooked veggies, we still need our nutrients.

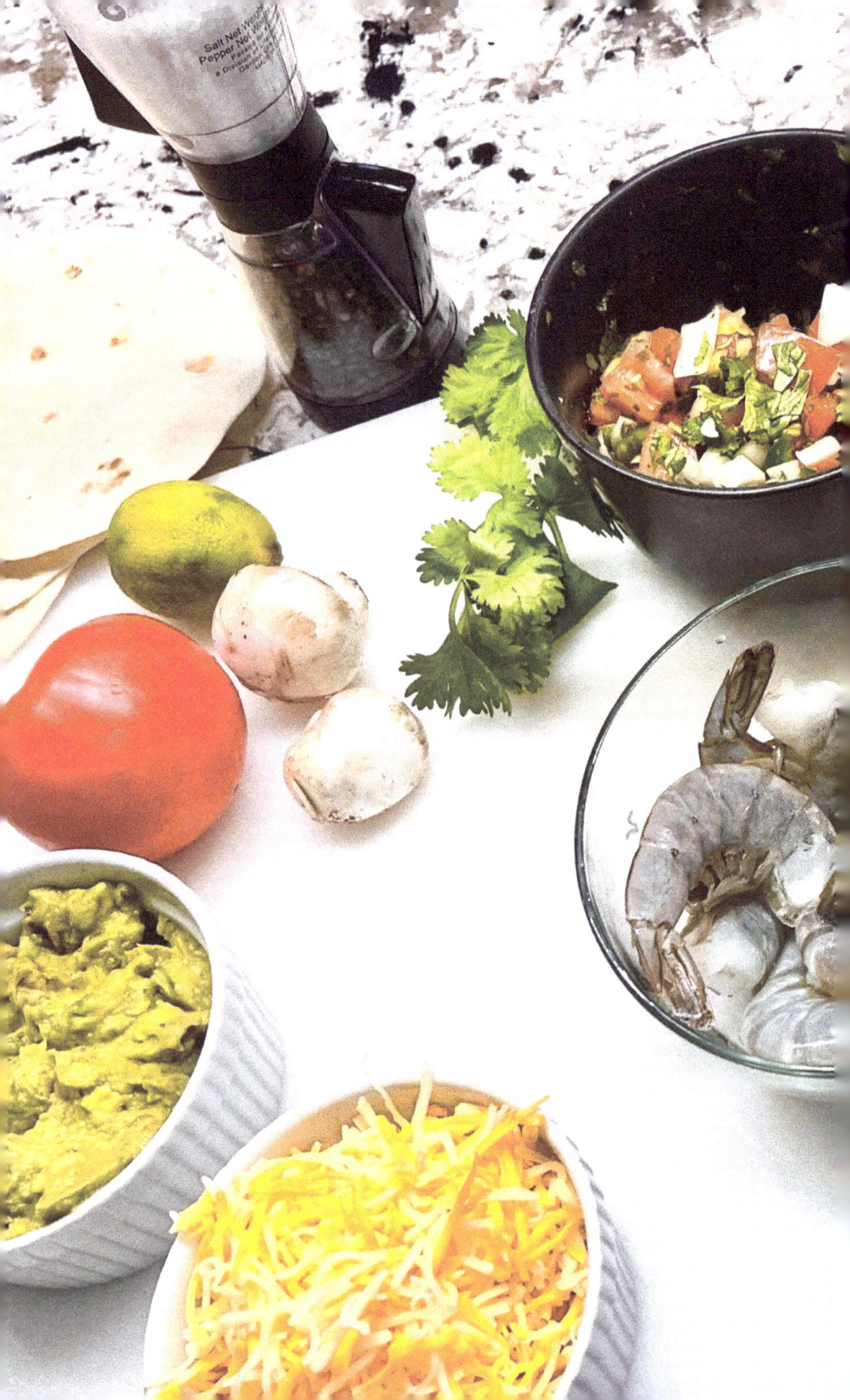

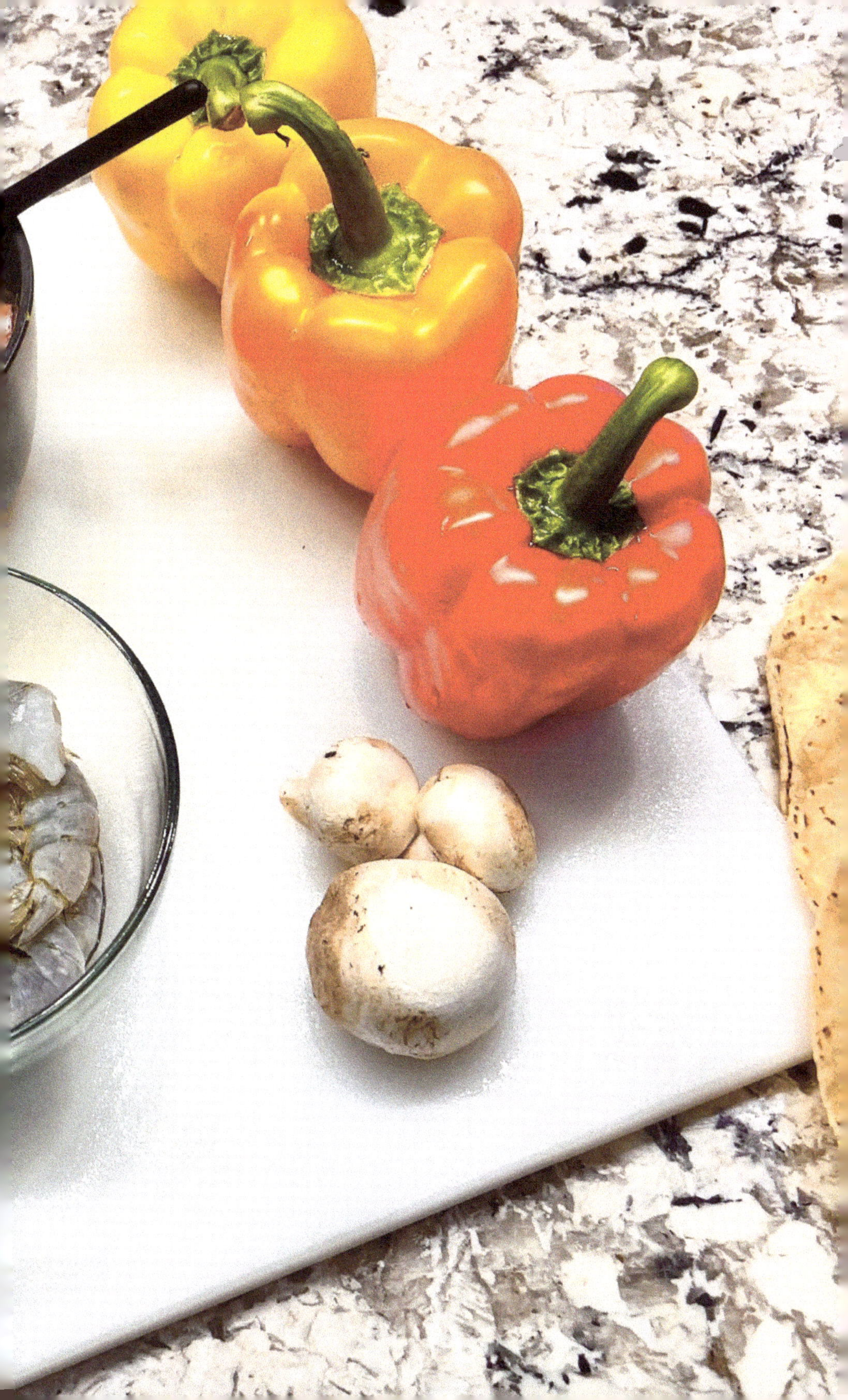

GARLIC BUTTER SHRIMP QUESADILLA

Who said Tuesdays are made for tacos? Well I say 'let's throw some quesadillas up in that thang'. Try these easy shrimp quesadillas on ANY day of the week!

- 2 flour 8" tortillas (or corn 4.5" tortillas - your preference)
- 4 tbsp olive oil
- ¼ cup mushrooms, sliced
- 1 cup sliced bell peppers (red, green, yellow, orange)
- ¼ red onion
- 1 cup fresh broccoli flowers
- 1 tsp onion powder
- 1 tsp garlic powder
- 1 tsp onion and herb seasoning
- 6 raw shrimp (de-shelled, deveined and cleaned)
- 1 tsp black pepper
- 1 tsp garlic salt
- 1 tsp Old Bay seasoning
- 1 tsp Tony Chachere's Creole seasoning
- 1 packet Sazon seasoning
- 1 tsp soy sauce
- 1 tbsp garlic butter
- 1 tbsp minced garlic
- ⅓ cup Mexican blend shredded cheese

Warm 2 tablespoons of oil and saute broccoli flowers, onions, bell peppers and mushrooms in a medium saucepan for 10 minutes. While the veggies are cooking, season them with soy sauce, onion powder, garlic salt, pepper and onion and herb seasoning. Once the veggies have finished cooking, set them aside on warm heat.

Season both sides of the de-shelled and deveined shrimp with creole seasoning, Old Bay seasoning, Sazon packet, garlic salt and black pepper.

Heat 1 tablespoon of oil in a medium saucepan and add in the shrimp. Add in garlic butter and minced garlic and be sure to cook your shrimp on both sides for 4-6 minutes or until the shrimp is pink and curled. Slice the shrimp down the middle and add the veggies. Top with cheese and set aside on warm heat.

Warm remaining oil in a medium skillet and place your tortilla in the center. While the shell is warming, load your veggies and shrimp on half of the tortilla shell. Fold the shell and cook on each side for 30 seconds - 1 minute, or until golden brown.

SERVES

2

*For quesadillas using corn shells, follow the recipe for shrimp quesadillas, but use two shells instead. Don't fold, instead you will place a second shell directly on top and flip the shell until it is golden brown on both sides.

Once quesadillas have finished cooking, cut the shells into a triangular shaped wedge and top with shredded cheese. Serve with salsa, guacamole and sour cream. Enjoy!

Classiq Tip:

For veggie quesadilla, simply omit the shrimp.

MOUTH WATERING ZUCCHINI BOATS (GF) (VG)

Who would've thought that loading veggies on top of veggies would taste so darn good? Well, let me be the first to tell you that this dish is like heaven on earth. Prepare your tastebuds for a light and refreshing meal. Take my word for it and check out this recipe below:

- 1 tbsp roasted garlic and herb seasoning
- 2 cups Gardein veggie crumbles
- 2 tbsp olive oil
- 1 tbsp soy sauce
- ⅓ cup mushrooms, diced
- ½ yellow bell pepper, diced
- ½ red bell pepper, diced
- ¼ cup onions, diced
- 1 tbsp onion powder
- 1 tbsp garlic salt
- 1 tsp sea salt
- 2 cups of your fav spaghetti sauce
- 1 tbsp sriracha
- ⅓ cup brown sugar
- ¼ cup Mexican blend shredded cheese

Preheat oven to 325 degrees

Slice the zucchini horizontally about ⅓ inch thick. You should be able to get 3-4 slices ("boats") from one large zucchini. Place zucchini slices in a pyrex pan and add olive oil. Bake Zucchini for 8-10 minutes. Remove the Zucchini and carve out ½ an inch from the middle of the boat. Be careful not to go too deep into the Zucchini slice.

Heat olive oil in a large skillet over low heat and add diced bell peppers, onions and mushrooms. While veggies are cooking for about 5 minutes, season them with soy sauce, garlic salt, black pepper, sea salt, onion powder, garlic and herb seasoning. Next add in the veggie crumble and cook for an additional 10 minutes.

While your veggie crumble contents are cooking, heat up spaghetti sauce on med-high in a medium pot. Next, stir in brown sugar and sriracha. Warm until sauce starts to boil. Once your sauce is nice and hot, add in your veggie crumble content and cook for 2-3 minutes.

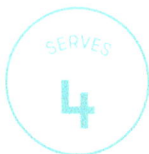

SERVES

4

Take zucchini boats out and top them off with the veggie crumble sauce. Sprinkle Mexican shredded cheese on top of the zucchini boats and bake for an additional 2-3 minutes or until the cheese is melted.

LEMON CRUSTED SEASONED SHRIMP (GF)

Prepare your mouth to water as you bite down into this juicy and flavorful shrimp. This is one of my favorites to cook. It's fairly easy to throw together and can be paired with almost anything. Bae Bae, these are so good that I bet you can't eat just one! Dare you to try em'!

- 6 fresh, raw shrimp (de-shelled, deveined and cleaned)
- ¼ cup Aldenis GF bread crumbs
- 1 tbsp olive oil
- 1 tsp roasted garlic and herb seasoning
- 1 tsp lemon juice
- 1 tsp minced garlic
- 1 tsp black pepper
- 1 tbsp garlic salt
- 1 tbsp Old Bay Seasoning
- 1 tbsp Tony Chachere's Creole seasoning
- 1 tsp parsley

After shrimp is thoroughly de-shelled, deveined and rinsed, season shrimp with pepper, garlic salt, old bay seasoning, Creole seasoning, and garlic and herb seasoning.

Coat the bottom of the skillet, heat olive oil, lemon juice and minced garlic occasionally stirring. Lightly coat each shrimp on both sides with breadcrumbs and place in oil to pan sear. Cook for 1-2 minutes on each side or until shrimp are pink and curled. Top with parsley!

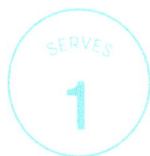

SERVES

1

Classiq Tip:

De-shell, Devein & Clean

- De-shelling shrimp: Hold the shrimp at the last segment before the tail, then pull off the rest of the shell, working from the underside to the top of the shrimp.

- Deveining shrimp: Hold the tail of the shrimp and use a sharp knife to slice the back of the shrimp, exposing the digestive tract (dark thread like structure). Be sure to pull the tract entirely out of the shrimp.

- Cleaning shrimp: In a large bowl, cover the unthawed shrimp with cold water and add in a tablespoon of apple cider vinegar and swoosh around.

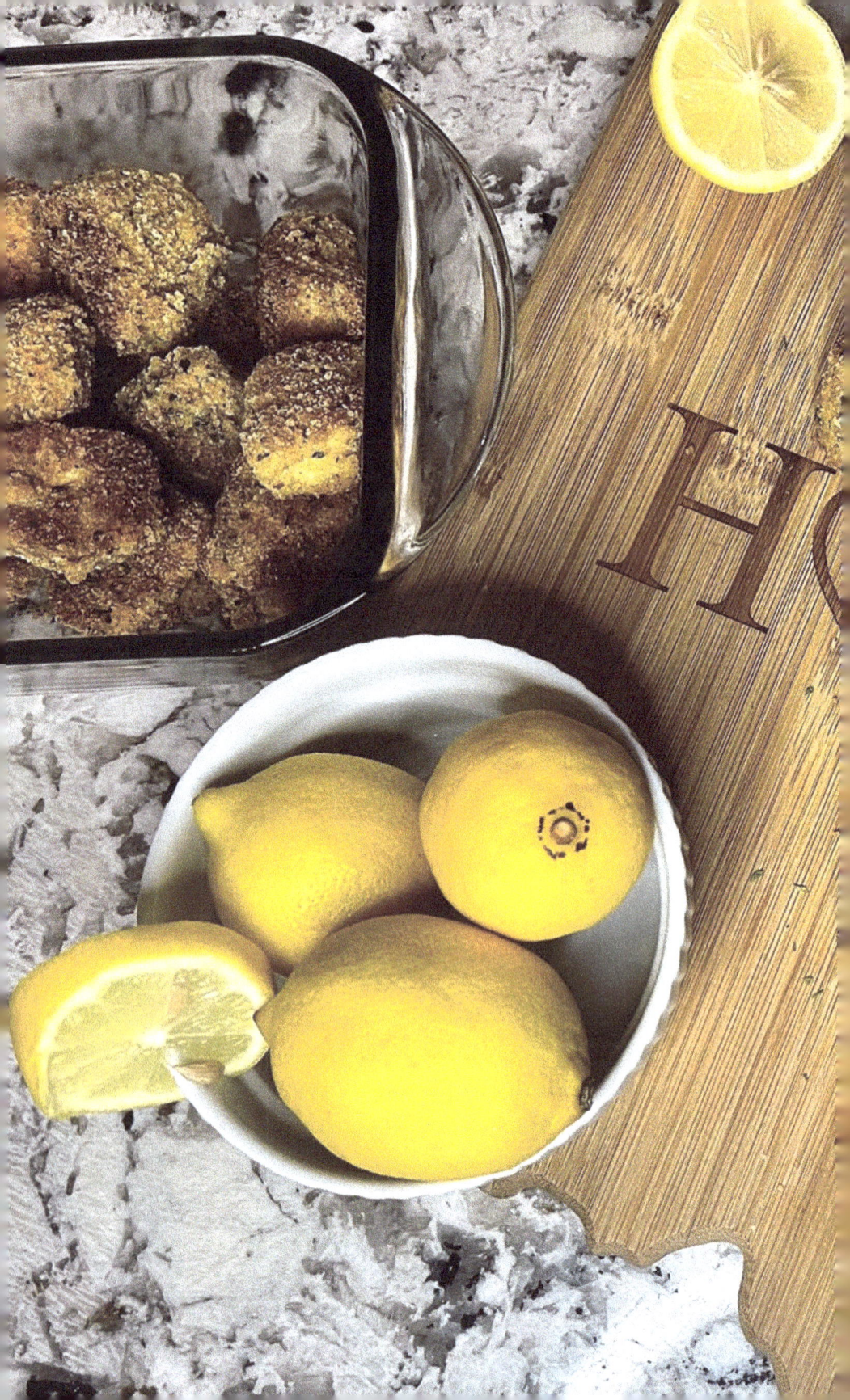

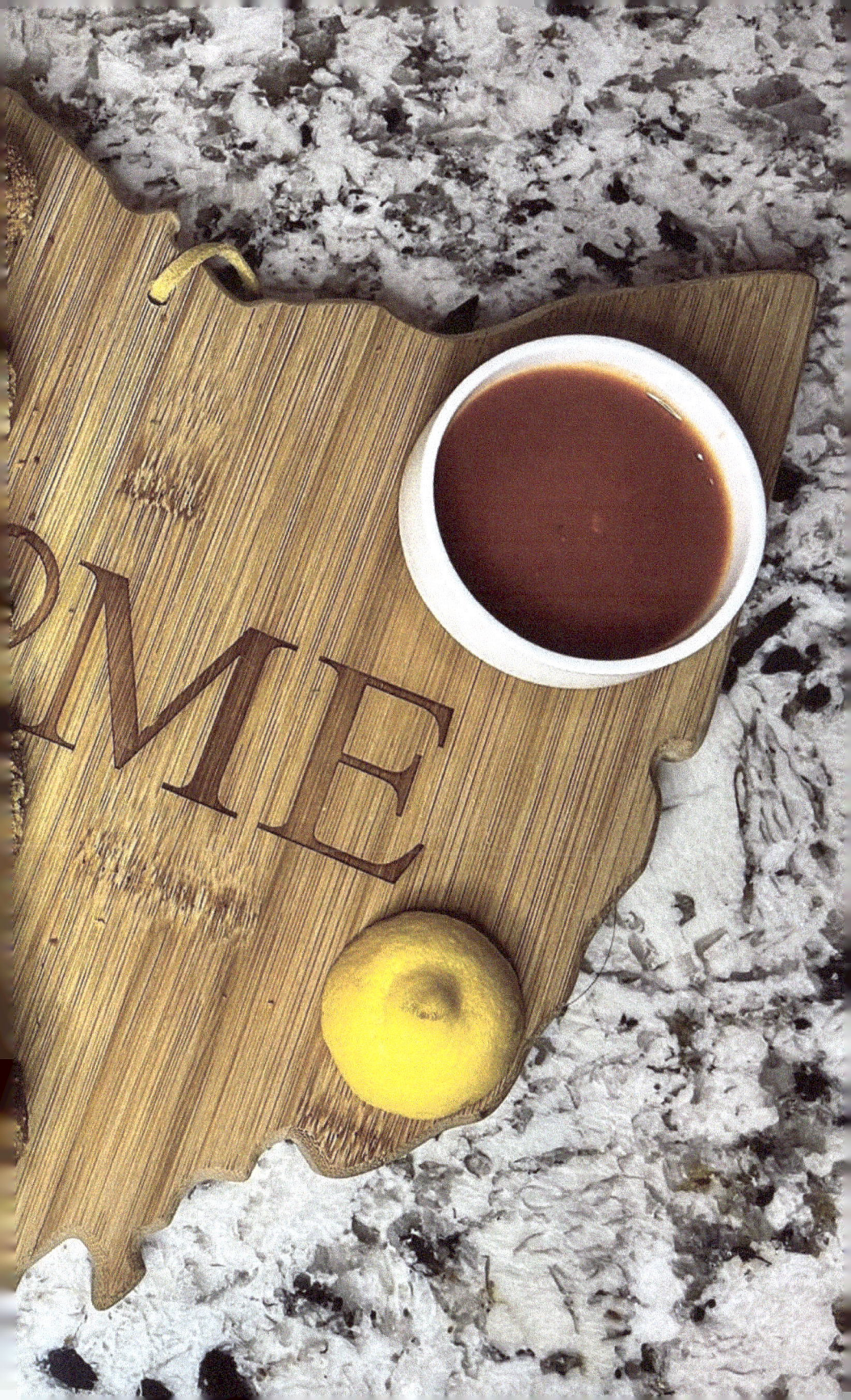

SAVORY SALMON NUGGETS (GF)

Back by popular demand!! These are dynamite and def worth every minute it takes to cook these to perfection. This recipe is by far the fans favorite. I guarantee you won't be disappointed.

- 2 fresh raw salmon filets (skinless and boneless)
- 1 cup Aldenis GF breadcrumbs
- 3 eggs, large
- 1 cup GF flour
- 1 cup GF plain panko
- 1 tbsp olive oil
- 1 tbsp roasted garlic and herb seasoning
- 1 tbsp garlic salt
- 1 tbsp black pepper
- 1 tbsp Old Bay seasoning
- 1 tbsp Tony Chachere's seasoning
- ½ packet Sazon seasoning
- 2 tbsp garlic butter
- 1 tsp parsley
- hot sauce (optional)
- 1 tbsp Jammin' Salmon

Preheat oven to 350 degrees

Whisk three eggs in a bowl. Mix flour and panko seasoning together in a bowl and place breadcrumbs in a separate bowl. Set the three bowls aside.

Cut the salmon into bite sized nuggets (about 1 ½ x 1 ½ inches). Season the nuggets with Old Bay, Tony Chachere's, Sazon, garlic salt, Jammin' Salmon, garlic and herb seasoning and black pepper. After you season the nuggets, dip them into the flour and panko mixture, then the whisked eggs, and lastly the breadcrumbs. Be sure to fully cover the nuggets in all three mixtures.

Heat olive oil and garlic butter in a large skillet. Place 10-12 nuggets in the skillet and pan sear each side for about 1-2 minutes or until nuggets form a flaky outer layer crust.

Place salmon nuggets on a lightly oiled baking sheet and cook thoroughly for 8-10 minutes. Top with parsley and serve with hot sauce.

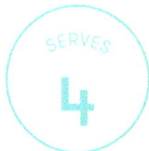

SERVES
4

Classiq Tip:

To warm up, reheat in the oven at 350 degrees for 5-10 minutes or in the air fryer at 400 degrees for 3 minutes. The microwave softens the batter and isn't very tasty.

PEPPERED "STEAK" ON A BED OF RICE (GF) (VG)

Growing up, my family loved eating steak. I remember the sound of my mom beating the meat and the smell of the steaks marinating the night before she cooked them. Well this is my spin on that juicy steak except mine is vegetarian of course. Today, we're pairing it with white rice and a creamy gluten free gravy. You are definitely in for a treat.

- 2 large portabella mushrooms, sliced
- 1 cup white rice, uncooked
- 1 tbsp butter
- 1 large green pepper, sliced
- 1 tbsp Italian blend seasoning
- 1 tbsp black pepper
- 2 tbsp salt
- 1 small onion, diced
- 1 tbsp minced garlic
- 1 tbsp garlic powder
- 1 tbsp onion powder
- 1 pack GF Brown Gravy (I use Pioneer brand)
- 2 cups vegetable broth
- 1 tsp dried basil

Rice:

Boil white rice for 10 minutes on medium in a medium pot. Then drain and place rice in a small bowl. Next, mix in butter and season with salt and black pepper and set aside.

Warm olive oil in a medium skillet and add in the onion, mushrooms, and bell pepper. While the veggies are sauteing, season with minced garlic, onion powder, garlic powder, black pepper, and Italian blend seasoning. Cook for 8-10 minutes or until the veggies have softened and set aside.

Boil 1 ½ cup of vegetable broth. Blend the gravy mix in with the remaining ½ cup of cool vegetable broth in a medium bowl. Whisk the contents together until the mixture is lump free. Then pour the gravy mix into the boiling broth and whisk until the gravy thickens.

Plate the rice and add veggies directly on top. Pour gravy on top of the rice, veggies and mushrooms. Garnish with basil and enjoy!

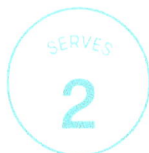

SERVES

2

Classiq Tip:

Once wet, mushrooms are nearly impossible to fully dry so don't bother. Instead, use a dry cloth to clean the excess debris.

66

Remember to
clean your seafood
& veggies

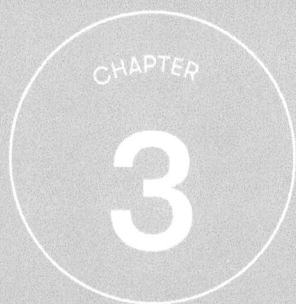

IT'S NEVER TOO LATE

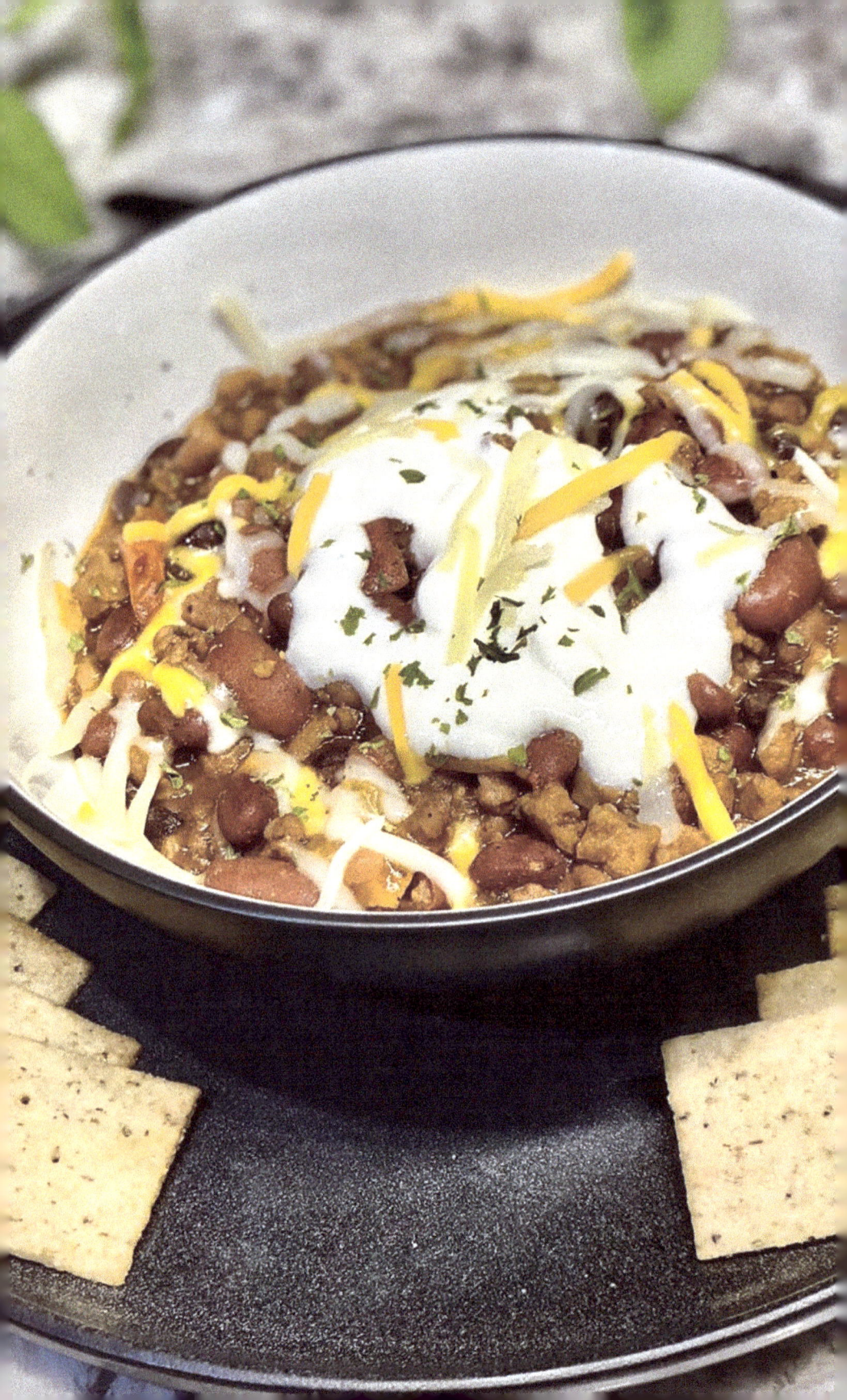

ALMOST VEGAN CHILI (GF) (VG)

Let's get into this chili chile (LOL). No really, this chili is a gift made from above! Its burst of flavorful beans and juicy sauces will have you wanting more. It's a perfect blend of tangy, spicy and sweet and gives you such a rush that you won't know what hit you. I honestly don't know how else to describe it. JUST GO MAKE THE DARN CHILI :-)

- 1 can kidney beans (15.5 oz) drained and rinsed
- 1 can black beans (15.5 oz) drained and rinsed
- 1 can chili beans (16 oz) drained and rinsed
- 1 can baked beans (28 oz), vegetarian
- 1 can fire roasted diced tomatoes (14.5 oz)
- 1 medium tomato, diced
- 1 packet, GF chili seasoning mix (I use McCormick brand)
- 1 red onion
- ⅓ green bell pepper, ⅓ red bell pepper, ⅓ yellow bell pepper
- 1 tbsp GF soy sauce
- 3 tbsp olive oil
- 1 tbsp of tomato paste
- 1 tsp liquid smoke
- 1 ½ cup vegetable broth
- 13.7 oz of your fav plant-based ground beef (I use Gardein)
- 1 tbsp brown sugar
- 1 tsp cumin
- 1 tbsp chili powder
- 1 tbsp onion powder
- 1 tbsp garlic powder
- 1 tbsp garlic salt
- 1 tbsp black pepper
- 1 tbsp roasted garlic and herb seasoning
- 2 rosemary leaves

SERVES
10

Set your slow cooker on high. While it's warming, dice the bell peppers and red onion.

Place kidney, chili, black and baked beans in the slow cooker. Add a cup of vegetable broth, canned tomatoes and tomato paste and allow the beans to cook for 30 minutes while you prepare the other ingredients.

Warm oil on medium and saute the plant-based ground beef, onions and bell peppers for 8-10 minutes in a large skillet. Season with onion powder, chili seasoning, chili powder, garlic powder, pepper, soy sauce, liquid smoke and roasted garlic and herb seasoning. Once the ingredients are done, add to the slow cooker and give it a good stir. Add in the remaining vegetable broth, brown sugar, and rosemary leaves and stir well. Cover the chili and continue to cook on high for 4-5 hours or until the beans are soft. In a bowl, top the chili off with cheese, sour cream and cilantro. Enjoy!

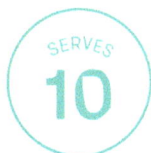

Classiq Tip:

For a thicker consistency, take a cup of the chili and blend/grind the contents for 10-15 sec. Add the blended chili back into the slow cooker and mix.

"

Anyone who says
they don't like Chili,
lied!

CREAMY SPINACH STUFFED SALMON (GF)

Listen honey, this dish tastes as good as it sounds. Creamy spinach, flaky salmon, parmesan cheese... um um um! If you need a recipe that will impress "that special someone" and have them thinking you've been in the kitchen since the birds started chirping, baby this is it!

- 5 fresh salmon filets (skinless, boneless)
- 9 ozs fresh spinach
- 8 ozs soft cream cheese
- 1 cup shredded parmesan cheese
- 2 tsp minced garlic
- 2 tsp salt
- 2 tsp black pepper
- 1 tbsp Tony's Chachere creole seasoning
- 1 tsp onion powder
- 2 tsp GF soy sauce
- 1 tbsp garlic salt
- 1 tbsp onion and herb seasoning
- 1 tsp Italian blend seasoning
- 2 tsp olive oil

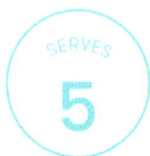

SERVES

5

Preheat the oven to 325 degrees

Start by adding 1 tbsp of olive oil in a medium skillet on low to medium and saute your spinach. Toss in garlic salt, soy sauce, onion powder, Italian blend seasoning and black pepper. Cook spinach until the leaves shrink and then drain.

Whisk together the cream cheese, shredded parmesan, minced garlic, salt, pepper and sauteed spinach in a large bowl until all ingredients are blended. Set the "stuffing" or spinach mixture aside.

Place the filets on a large cutting board and cut 2" slits in the center of each fillet so both top and bottom sections make an even pocket. Next, season the salmon on both sides with salt, pepper, Tony's creole seasoning, and onion and herb seasoning. Then, stuff 1-2 tablespoons of the spinach mixture into the pockets. Avoid overstuffing the salmon to prevent the contents from oozing out while cooking.

Heat the remaining oil in a large skillet on medium and sear both sides of the salmon for 1-2 minutes. Once you have obtained a flaky crust-like layer on each side, place the stuffed salmon on a greased baking sheet and bake for 10-15 minutes. Be sure to place the baking sheet on the top rack. Allow the salmon to cool before plating. Enjoy!

Classiq Tip:

- ALWAYS USE FRESH SPINACH!
- Refrigerate any leftover spinach mixture and you'll have an amazing spinach dip!

GUILT-FREE ZUCCHINI SPAGHETTI (GF) (VG) (V)

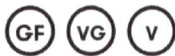

This healthy recipe is surprisingly filling, but will leave you feeling lite. Crazy, right! It's safe to serve this meal at any function because everyone enjoys it, especially my vegan lovers!

- 1 container zucchini noodles (buy or make 12 ozs. I use Del Monte's brand)
- 13.7 ozs of your fav plant-based ground beef (I use Gardein)
- ⅓ cup mushrooms
- ¼ yellow bell pepper, ¼ red bell pepper, ¼ orange bell pepper
- 2 tbsp olive oil
- ⅓ onion
- 3 large tomatoes (peeled)
- 1 can (6 oz) tomato paste
- 1 tbsp onion powder
- 1 tbsp garlic powder
- 1 tsp soy sauce
- 1 tbsp black pepper
- 1 tbsp sea salt
- 1 tbsp Italian medley seasoning blend
- 1 tbsp roasted garlic and herb seasoning
- 1 tsp parsley
- 1 tbsp minced garlic
- ¼ cup of brown sugar
- 1 tsp lemon juice

Dice bell peppers and onions and cut off all stems from tomatoes. In lukewarm water, rinse zucchini noodles off and then place to the side to allow the noodles to dry. Zucchini typically holds water for a while so you may even want to pat them with a napkin.

Saute onions, bell peppers and mushrooms with olive oil, black pepper, onion powder and half the sea salt. While your veggies are cooking add in your plant-based ground beef and season with Italian medley seasoning, garlic powder, and then set aside.

Sauce:

Peel tomatoes and blend in a food processor until they appear to have a thick consistency. In a medium pot cook blended tomatoes on medium for 10 minutes. Add in tomato paste, onion garlic and herb seasoning, minced garlic, brown sugar, and lemon juice.

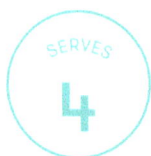

SERVES

4

Allow sauce to come to a boil and then add in your veggies and plant-based ground beef mixture. Cook for an additional 5 minutes on low.

Heat olive oil on low to medium in a medium skillet. Place the zucchini noodles in the skillet and let them cook for 5-8 minutes. While the noodles are cooking, season them with the remaining sea salt and pepper. Plate noodles and pour your desired amount of sauce on top. Enjoy!

Classiq Tip:

- I use a potato peeler to peel tomatoes. You could always boil the tomatoes to soften and easily peel with your hands or a knife.
- This meal is delicious with or without plant-based meat.

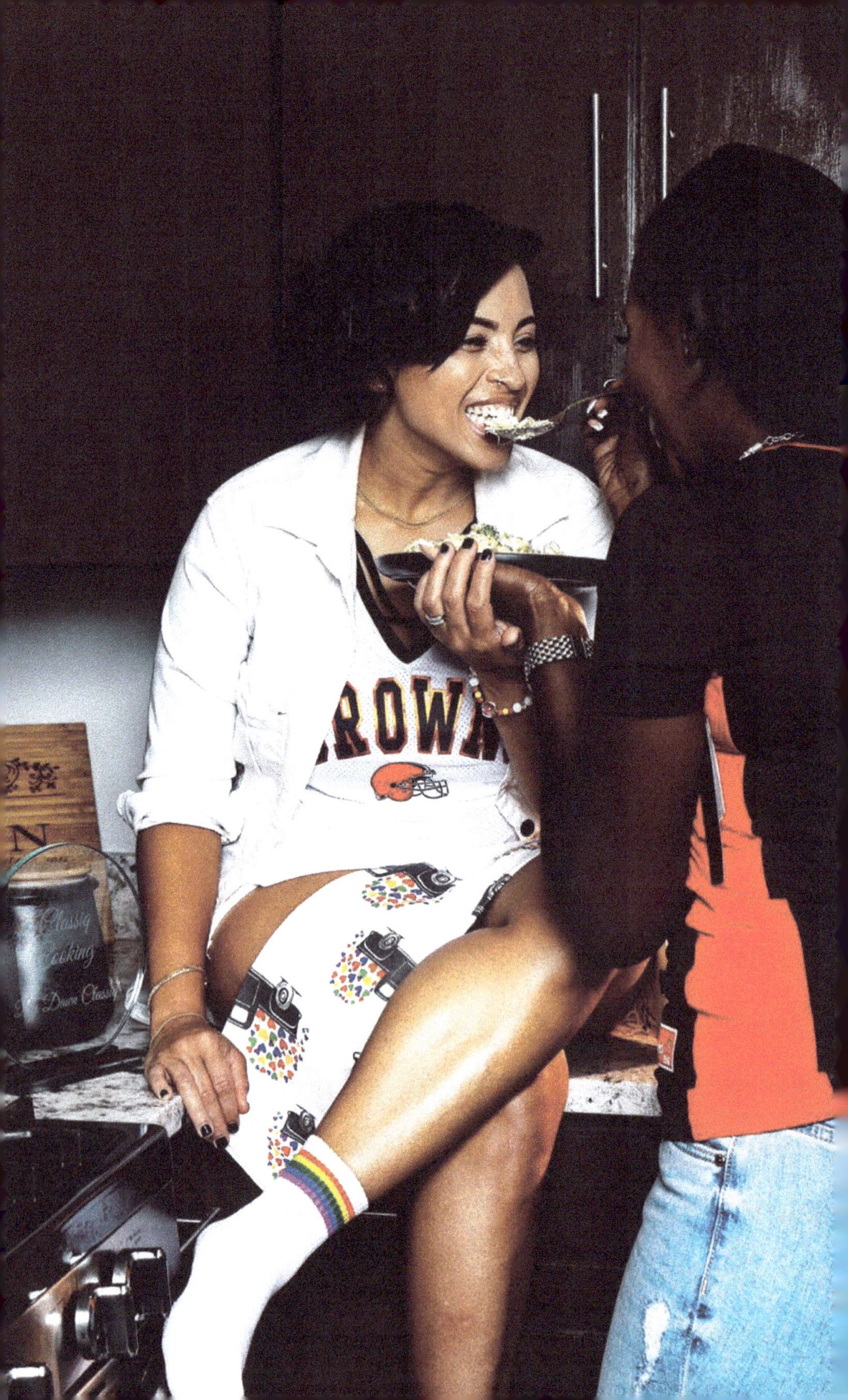
ROWN

RICH & GOOEY
VEGETABLE ALFREDO (GF) (VG)

Now I know I told you the Savory Salmon Nuggets were the fan favorite, but I can't lie, this may be the runner up. Once you make this Veggie Alfredo, your friends and family will have you cooking this dish for every birthday celebration, baby shower and national holiday! Dare to share!

- 1 box penne noodles, GF (16 oz)
- 2 ½ cups mushrooms
- ½ onion
- 12 oz bag of fresh broccoli
- 1 stick of butter
- 2 tbsp olive oil
- 16 oz heavy whipping cream
- 8 oz soft cream cheese
- 1 ½ cups shredded parmesan cheese
- ½ cup shredded mozzarella cheese
- 1 tbsp GF soy sauce
- 2 tbsp minced garlic
- 2 tbsp garlic salt
- 1 tbsp garlic powder
- 2 tbsp onion powder
- 1 tbsp onion and herb seasoning
- 2 tbsp black pepper
- 1 tbsp parsley
- 2 tbsp salt

SERVES
10

Preheat oven to 400 degrees. Cut off broccoli stalks and discard and finely slice the mushrooms.

Boil 3 ½ cups of water in a large pot and add 1 tbsp of salt to the water. This helps give the pasta some flavor. Next, stir in penne noodles. Allow noodles to boil for 8-10 minutes. Once noodles are cooked, drain and empty contents into a pyrex pan.

Boil 3 cups of water in a large pot and then place the broccoli in the boiled water. Cook for 5 minutes. Add in the remaining salt, a tbsp of pepper and a tbsp of butter. Once the broccoli has finished cooking, drain and pour broccoli into the pyrex pan with the noodles.

Warm the olive oil in a small skillet on low and saute mushroom and onions for 8 minutes. Season with soy sauce, garlic salt, pepper and onion and herb seasoning. Once your mushrooms and onions are cooked, place them in the pyrex pan with the noodles and broccoli.

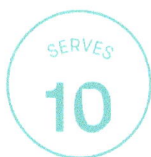

Alfredo sauce:

In a large pot, whisk in the heavy whipping cream, cream cheese, shredded parmesan cheese, stick of butter and minced garlic and heat on warm. Allow the contents to simmer and whisk in your black pepper, garlic powder, onion powder and garlic salt. Stir for 8-10 minutes.

Once the sauce has thickened, pour it into the pyrex pan with all other ingredients and mix thoroughly. Top off with mozzarella cheese then place the pan in the oven on the middle rack for 15-20 minutes or until the cheese has melted and is golden brown. Lastly, take alfredo out and top off with parsley. Allow veggie alfredo to cool before serving. Enjoy!

Classiq Tip:

Make sure the water is boiling BEFORE adding in pasta and broccoli. The intense heat helps to "set" the outside of the pasta, which prevents the pasta from sticking. Boiling the water first helps the broccoli produce a crisp, yet tender texture. You'll thank me later!

GLUTEN - FREE MEATLESS MEATLOAF SUB ⓋⒼ

Let's be honest, who doesn't love a good meatball sub? I know I do! And get this, it's not even real meat. This meatloaf sub has a twist on the meatballs. This creation is another gift from above... And the sauce is to die for! This is simply one of my favorite recipe remixes.

- 8 of your fav Italian Subs or GF buns (I use Schwebel's brand)
- 4 tbsp olive oil
- 13.7 oz of your fav plant-based ground beef, unthawed (I use Beyond Beef plant-based ground)
- ⅓ green bell pepper
- ½ onion, chopped
- 1 tbsp GF soy sauce
- 1 tbsp onion powder
- 1½ tbsp black pepper
- 1 tbsp sea salt
- 1 cup Aldenis GF breadcrumbs
- 1 cup uncooked white rice (I use boil-in-bag Success brand)
- 1 tsp salt
- 2 tbsp butter
- 1 egg
- 2 tbsp brown sugar
- 1 tbsp hot sauce
- 1 tbsp ketchup
- 1 cup almond milk
- 1 tbsp liquid smoke
- 1 cup Diya pepper jack cheese

Preheat the oven to 350 degrees and dice the onion and green pepper.

Rice:
Boil 3 cups of water in a medium pot and then add in one bag of rice (or 1 cup of rice). Cook on medium for 10 minutes. Once the rice is cooked, use a small mixing bowl to combine rice, butter, salt and pepper.

Meatloaf:
In a mixing bowl, place the unthawed plant-based meat, cooked rice, diced peppers, onions, egg, breadcrumbs, liquid smoke, almond milk, ketchup, onion powder, sea salt and pepper. Wear a glove to knead all ingredients together until the flavors are thoroughly mixed in and contents begin to form a solid loaf.

Lightly oil a loaf pan with olive oil and place all contents in the pan to ensure that the "meat" stays firm and in the shape of a loaf.

Sauce:

In a mixing bowl whisk together brown sugar, ketchup and hot sauce until the sauce appears loose and sticky.

Layer a thick coat of the sauce on top of the meatloaf before placing the pan in the oven, on the top rack. Bake for 45 minutes. When the meatloaf has finished cooking, allow it to set and cool and then slice the "meat" into about one inch thick slices. Set this aside while you toast your sub.

Toast the sub in a small non-stick skillet with butter on low for 3 minutes or until golden brown. Once you plate the sub, coat the inner surfaces of your sub with your favorite condiments. I use a thin layer of sriracha mayo and a little Miracle whip.

Add a slice of the meat loaf and top it off with a sprinkle of pepper jack cheese. Drizzle additional sauce if desired. Enjoy!

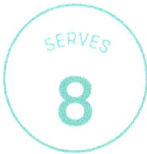

SERVES
8

Classiq Tip:

For a healthier option, ditch the bread and pair this yummy meatloaf with our Garlic Parmesan Asparagus.

RED BEANS & QUINOA (GF) (VG)

Six words:

Better. Than. Red. Beans. And. Rice.

- 3 cans red kidney beans (drained and rinsed)
- 1 cup quinoa (boil-in-bag Success brand)
- 3 cups vegetable broth
- 2 cups water
- 1 tbsp roasted garlic and herb seasoning
- 1 tbsp garlic salt
- 1 tbsp minced garlic
- 1 tbsp black pepper
- ⅓ onion
- ½ green bell pepper
- 1 tsp parsley
- 2 bay leaves
- 1 tsp dried basil
- 1 tsp sage
- 1 tbsp salt
- 2 tbsp olive oil
- 2 tbsp butter
- 1 tsp cayenne pepper
- 1 tbsp Jamaican seasoning

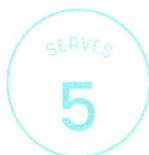

SERVES

5

Heat half the vegetable broth in a medium pot on medium for 3 minutes or until the broth starts to boil. Turn your slow cooker on high and add in the remaining broth, beans, and bay leaves and cook for 2 to 3 hours or until beans are soft. Cover beans with a lid.

Dice onion and bell pepper and set aside. Season the beans with black pepper, salt, cayenne pepper, sage, basil, and Jamaican seasoning while it's in the slow cooker and mix well. Pour the boiling broth into the slow cooker and stir.

Heat olive oil in a medium skillet and saute onions and bell peppers on low-medium. Season with garlic and herb seasoning, minced garlic, garlic salt and black pepper for 5-10 minutes. Once veggies are cooked, add them into the slow cooker.

Boil 2 cups of water in a small pot and then add in the bag of quinoa and cook on medium for 10 minutes. Once the quinoa has cooked, combine butter, salt and black pepper in a small mixing bowl and stir ingredients together. Serve this dish in a glass bowl and Enjoy!

Classiq Tip:

Do not overcook the Quinoa. 10 MINUTES ONLY!!!

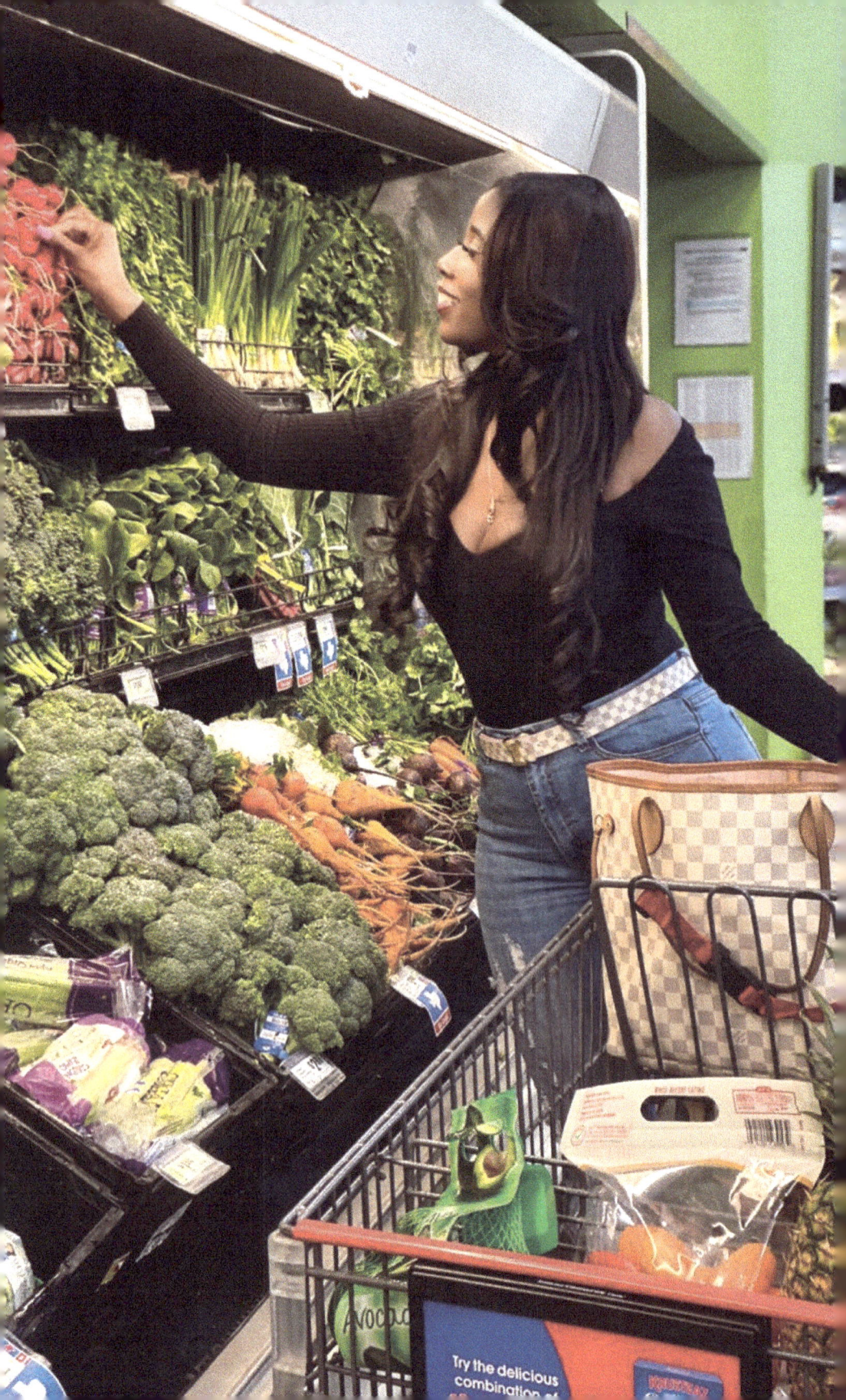

Strive each day to be
the best version of
yourself!

CHEESY STUFFED BELL PEPPERS (GF) (VG)

Okay, so the last time I cooked these stuffed bell peppers, my cousin requested for me to make it three weekends in a row... (Yeah, I know exactly what you're thinking). What can I say? They're yummy and delicious!

- 2 red bell peppers, 2 orange bell peppers, 2 yellow bell peppers (6 total)
- 2 cups white rice (boil-in-bag Success brand)
- 1½ cups mushrooms
- ½ onion
- 12oz bag of fresh broccoli
- 10 tbsp butter
- 2 tbsp olive oil
- 6 cups of water
- 16 ozs heavy whipping cream
- 8 ozs soft cream cheese
- 1½ cups shredded parmesan
- ½ cup mozzarella cheese
- 2 tbsp GF soy sauce
- 2 tbsp minced garlic
- 1 tbsp garlic salt
- 1 tbsp garlic powder
- 1 tbsp onion powder
- 1 tbsp black pepper
- 1 tsp parsley
- 2 tbsp salt

Preheat the oven to 350 degrees then cut the stalks from the broccoli and discard.

Dice onion and mushrooms. Then, slice off the top of the bell peppers and remove the seeds.

Coat the bottom of the pyrex pan with olive oil. Next, place the peppers in the pan and drizzle olive oil, a pinch of salt and black pepper on top. Then place the peppers in the oven on the top rack for 15-20 minutes or until bell peppers appear warped and soft. Take out and set aside.

Rice:
Boil 3 cups of water in a medium pot and then add in two bags of rice. Cook on medium for 10 minutes. Once the rice is cooked, use a large mixing bowl to combine rice, 2 tbsp of butter, a sprinkle of salt and pepper. Set rice aside.

Boil 3 cups of water in a large pot and then drop the broccoli in the boiled water and let cook for 5 minutes. Add in a tablespoon of salt, a tablespoon of black pepper and a tablespoon of butter. Once broccoli is done cooking, drain and pour broccoli into the mixing bowl with the rice.

Alfredo sauce:
In a large pot, whisk in the heavy whipping cream, cream cheese, shredded parmesan cheese, remaining 8 tbsp of butter and minced garlic on warm. Allow the contents to simmer and whisk in your black pepper, garlic powder, onion powder and garlic salt. Stir for 8-10 minutes.

Once the sauce has thickened, pour half of the sauce into the mixing bowl with the rice and mix all ingredients together. Fill each bell pepper with the rice and veggies mixture and top with the remaining sauce and mozzarella cheese. Place in the oven on the middle rack for 20 minutes or until the cheese has melted and has a golden brown layer. Top off with parsley and allow stuffed bell peppers to cool before serving. Enjoy!

SERVES
6-8

Classiq Tip:

Be sure to cook the bell peppers before stuffing them to ensure that they will be soft. There's nothing worse than a hard bell pepper with yummy insides.

"

Who says cooking has to be boring? Cooking can be fun, sexy and most importantly, classiq.

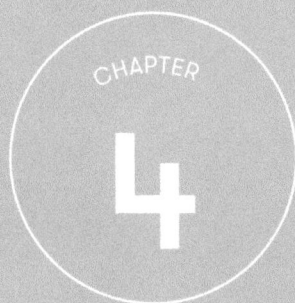

SOPHISTICATED SIDES

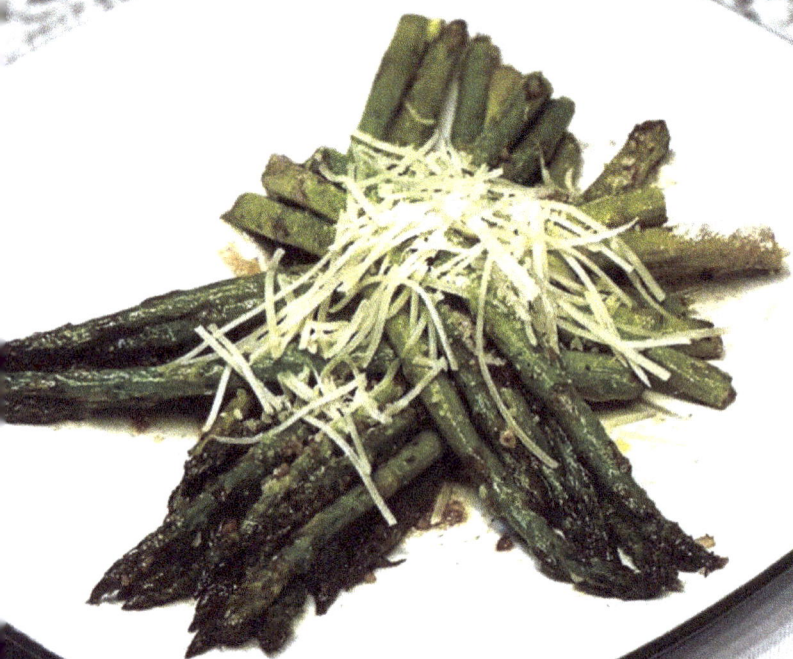

GARLIC PARMESAN ASPARAGUS (GF) (VG)

- 3 handfuls fresh asparagus
- ¼ cup shredded parmesan cheese
- ¼ cup grated parmesan cheese
- 1 tbsp minced garlic
- 1 tbsp garlic salt
- 1 tbsp black pepper
- 1 tbsp garlic powder
- 1 tbsp onion powder
- 1 tbsp onion and herb seasoning
- 3 tbsp olive oil

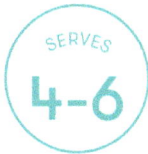

SERVES

4-6

Preheat the oven to 375 degrees.

Slice off the pale ends of the asparagus stalks. Lightly oil the bottom of a baking sheet and arrange the asparagus to form a single layer.

Season asparagus with garlic salt, pepper, garlic powder, onion powder, onion and herb seasoning and minced garlic.

Drizzle olive oil on top of the seasoned asparagus and place the baking sheet on the middle rack. Cook the asparagus for 15-20 minutes.

After the tips of the asparagus become brown, top the asparagus off with shredded and grated parmesan and bake for 5 more minutes or until the cheese has melted.

Classiq Tip:

Did you know that asparagus is used to treat bee stings and tooth aches? How about using asparagus to relieve you of a hangover? No? Try this hack next time you've had one-to-many.

GLAZED BROCCOLI AND CAULIFLOWER MEDLEY

(GF) (VG)

- 2 cups fresh broccoli
- 2 cups fresh cauliflower
- 3 tbsp Jamaican seasoning
- ¼ cup brown sugar
- 1 tbsp crushed red peppers (or red pepper flakes)
- 1 stick butter
- 1 tbsp salt
- 1 tbsp soy sauce, GF
- 1 tbsp black pepper
- 1 tbsp onion and herb seasoning
- 1 tbsp onion powder

SERVES

5

Preheat the oven to 375 degrees.

Cut off the stalk and florets of the broccoli and cauliflower and break apart the flowers. Then place the medley on a sheet of double duty aluminum foil.

Season the broccoli and cauliflower with brown sugar, Jamaican seasoning, salt, black pepper, red pepper flakes, onion powder, soy sauce and onion and herb seasoning. Mix well.

Place ¼ of butter in each corner of the foil and then seal and fold both ends closing the contents entirely. Take your fork and poke small holes in the top of the foil. Place the medley on a baking sheet, on the middle rack and cook for 20 -25 minutes. Enjoy!

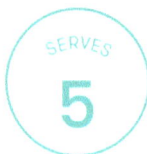

Classiq Tip:

Did you know?

- Broccoli was introduced to the United States in the 1800's by Italians!
- Cauliflower is a great source of Vitamin C.
- Try this recipe on the grill and the roasted flavors will have you in a summer mood.

BRUSSELS LIKE NO OTHER (GF) (VG)

- 4 cups fresh brussel sprouts
- 3 tbsp olive oil
- ¼ cup brown sugar
- 1 tbsp salt
- 1 tbsp black pepper
- 1 tbsp onion and herb seasoning
- 1 tbsp onion powder
- 1 tbsp table blend seasoning
- 1 tbsp soy sauce

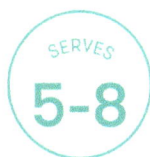

SERVES
5-8

Preheat the oven to 425 degrees.

Cut off the stems of the brussel sprouts. Slice brussel sprouts in half. Drizzle olive oil in a pyrex pan and place brussel sprouts flat in the pan.

Season the brussels sprouts with salt, pepper, onion and herb seasoning, onion powder, soy sauce and table blend seasoning and mix well.

Place brussel sprouts in the oven on the middle rack and cook for 25 minutes. Allow brussels to cool before serving. Enjoy!

Classiq Tip:

When selecting your brussel sprouts try to look for tightly wrapped sprouts, bright green color and firm stems.

STREET CORN (GF) (VG)

- 4 ears of corn
- ¼ cup sour cream
- ¼ cup mayonnaise
- ½ cup feta cheese
- 1 tsp minced garlic
- 1 lemon, juice
- 1 lime zest
- ¼ cup fresh cilantro
- ½ tsp chipotle seasoning
- 1 tsp chili powder

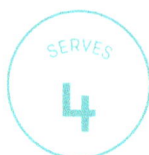

SERVES

4

Soak corn with husks on in cool water for 10 minutes before grilling.

Start your grill at 400 degrees or try to obtain a medium/high fire.

Place the corn on the grill, still with the husk on and cook for 12-15 minutes turning every 3-5 minutes. Once the corn is cooked, allow it to cool and remove the husk. Be sure to rinse off any excess corn silk.

In a small mixing bowl, mix in the sour cream, mayonnaise, feta cheese, minced garlic, lemon juice, zest of lime, chipotle seasoning and cilantro.

Coat each corn on the cob with the cheese mixture and sprinkle with chili powder. Lastly, top off the corn with another layer of feta cheese and cilantro and enjoy!

Classiq Tip:

If you don't have a grill or don't have the time to grill, set the oven on broil and cook each side for 6-8 minutes. This works like magic!

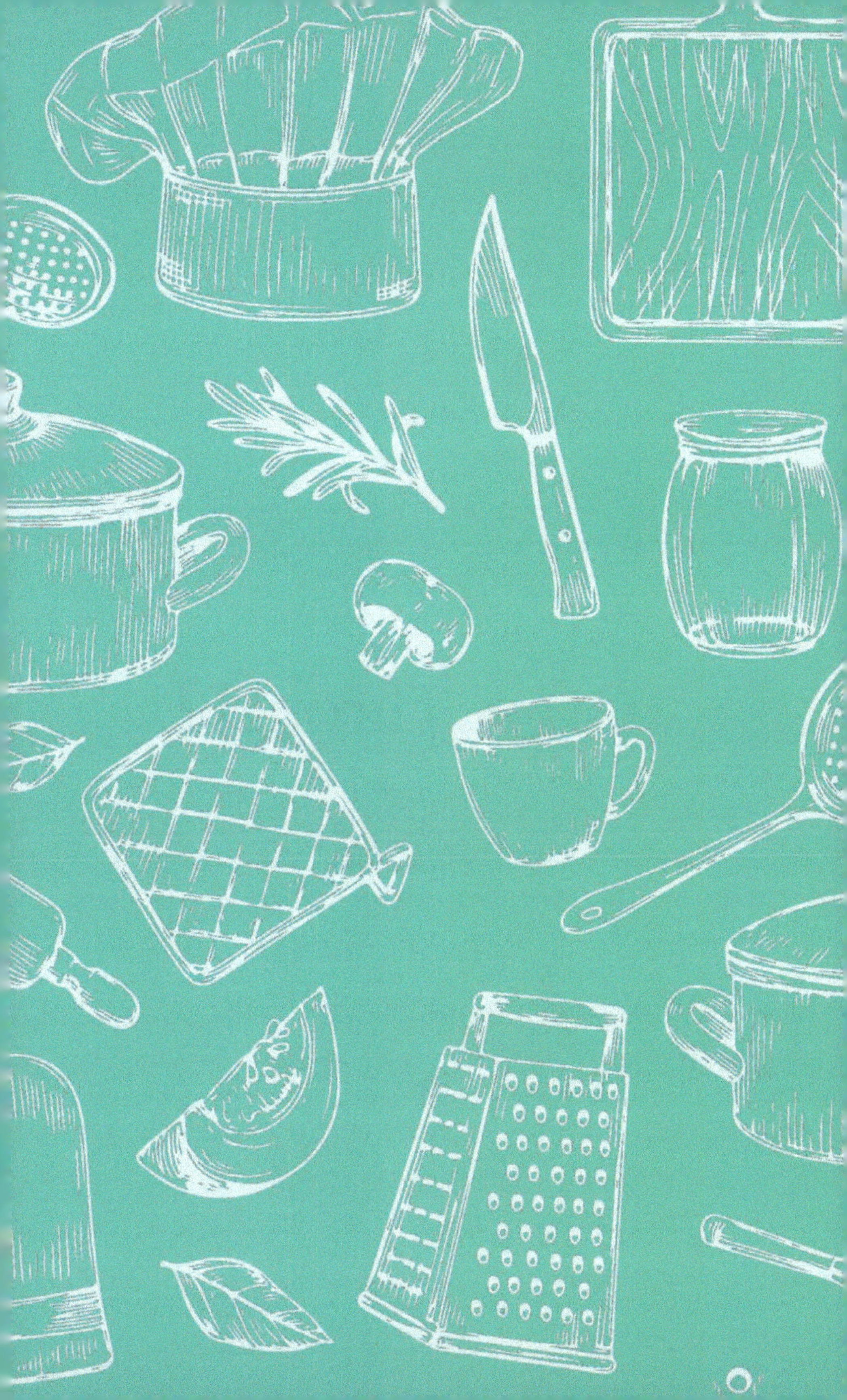

Come Through!

CHAPTER

5

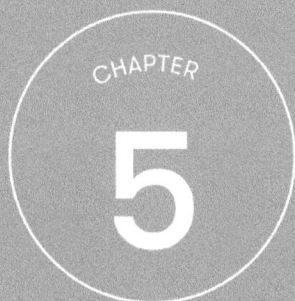

SLAYED SALADS

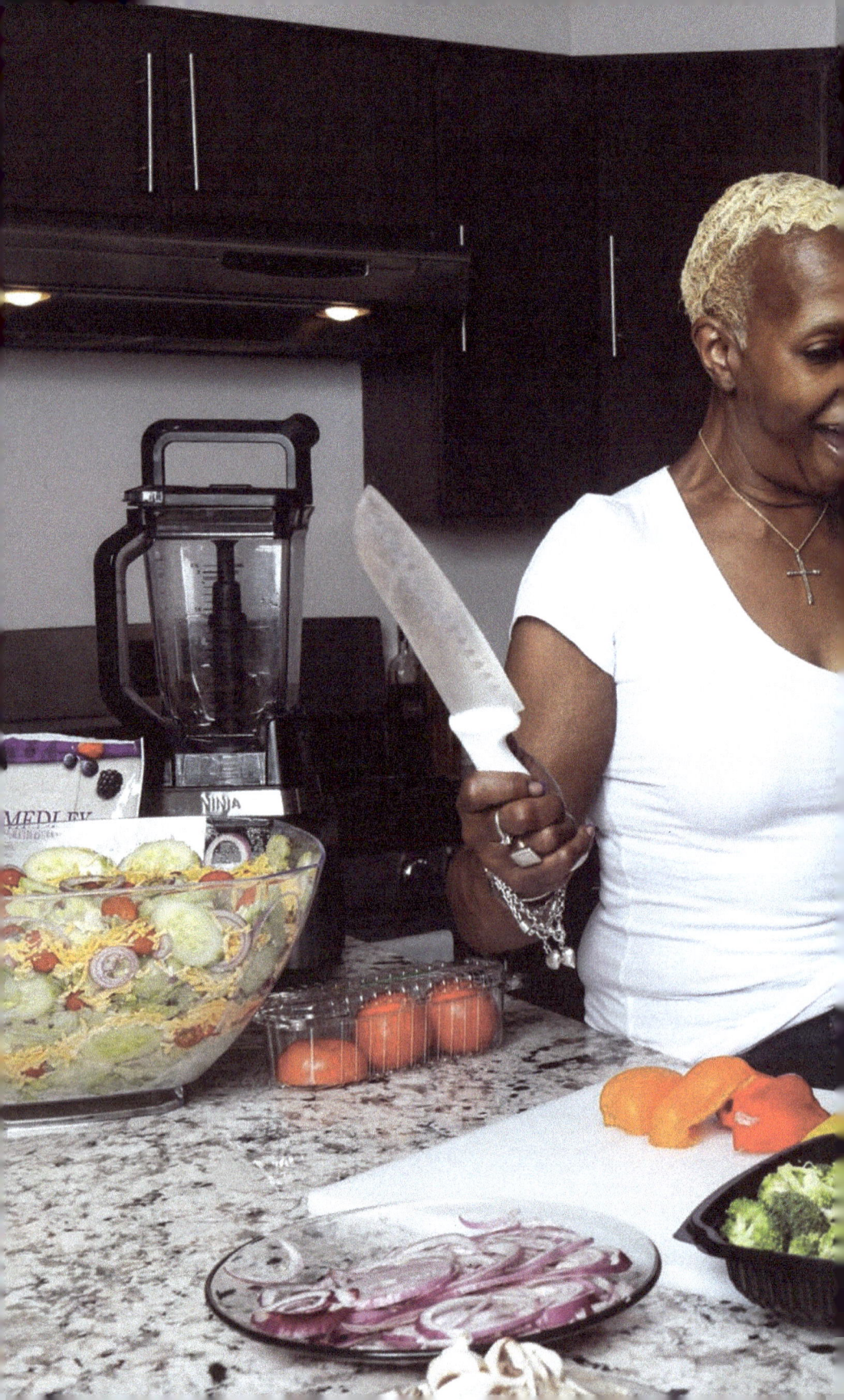

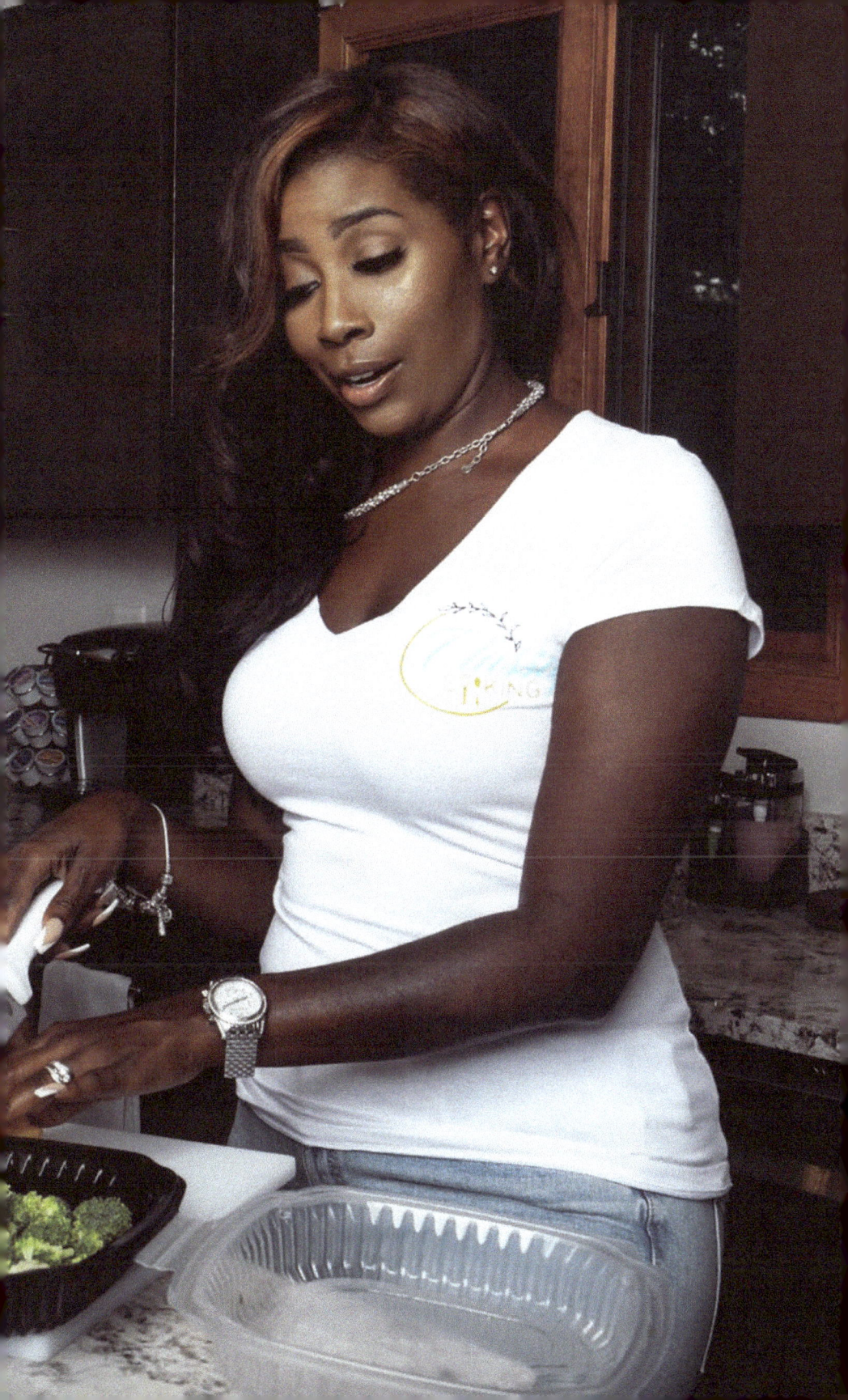

SOUTHWEST SALAD (VG)

- 2 cups Iceberg lettuce, chopped
- ⅓ cup sweet corn, canned
- ¼ cup black beans, canned
- ½ cup sweet red and orange bell peppers, sliced
- 2 tbsp onion, chopped
- ½ cup shredded Mexican cheese blend
- 1 tsp roasted garlic and herb seasoning
- 1 tsp taco seasoning
- 1 tsp onion powder
- ¼ cup tortilla strips
- 2 tbsp salt
- 2 tbsp black pepper
- 1 cup vegetable broth
- 2 tbsp olive oil
- 2 tbsp soy sauce

Saute bell peppers and onions in olive oil and soy sauce in a small skillet on medium. Then mix in the taco seasoning. Next, rinse and drain beans and corn.

Warm the corn in a saucepan on medium and add 1 tbsp salt and black pepper to taste. Next, boil the black beans in vegetable broth for 10-15 minutes or until the beans are softened. Season with onion powder and garlic and herb seasoning.

Rinse, dry and cut the iceberg lettuce and season lightly with 1 tbsp salt and black pepper. Next, combine all the ingredients in a medium bowl and top with shredded cheese and tortilla strips. Finish this salad off with your choice of salad dressing and enjoy!

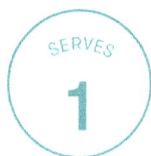

SERVES
1

Classiq Tip:

This salad pairs well with Southwest Chipotle salad dressing.

GARDEN SALAD (GF) (VG)

- 2 cups chopped romaine lettuce
- 2 cups water
- ¼ cup red onion, sliced
- ¼ cup halved cherry tomatoes
- ¼ cucumber
- ¼ cup croutons (optional)
- ¼ cup shredded sharp cheddar cheese
- 2 medium eggs, boiled
- 1 tsp salt
- 1 tsp black pepper

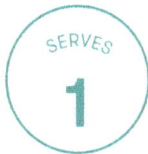

SERVES

1

Boil the eggs in two cups of water in a small pot on medium for 10-12 minutes. Remove the eggs with a spoon and allow them to cool before peeling. Peel off the shells under cold water and slice before setting aside.

Rinse, dry and cut the romaine lettuce and then lightly season with 1 tbsp salt and black pepper. Next, plate romaine lettuce first, then layer on your cucumber slices and cherry tomatoes. Finally add onions, eggs and croutons. Top off your salad with cheese and your choice of salad dressing and enjoy!

Classiq Tip:

This salad pairs well with an authentic ranch dressing.

“

Create a guilt-free
atmosphere.

SINFUL TREAT

DELIGHTFUL
BANANA PUDDING ⓖⒻ

Imagine the best banana pudding you ever had... Now imagine it tasting 100 times better, AND it's gluten free! This sinful treat will turn you from classiq to crazy in just one bite!

- 3 large overripe bananas, sliced
- 3 boxes GF shortbread cookies, (you can crumble if you want them finer I use Walkers GF pure butter shortbread brand)
- 14 ozs sweetened condensed milk
- 8 ozs cream cheese, soft
- 2 cups almond milk
- 5.1 oz box vanilla pudding, (I use Jell-O Brand)
- 3 tsp granulated sugar
- 2 cups heavy whipping cream
- 1½ tsp vanilla extract

SERVES
10-15

Use a chilled bowl to mix the heavy whipping cream, vanilla extract, and sugar together until whipped cream is formed. Set aside in the refrigerator to cool.

Combine the cream cheese and condensed milk with a hand mixer. Then mix almond milk and pudding together in a large bowl. Stir in the cream cheese mixture and continue mixing until the contents are smooth.

Add in two cups of the fresh whipped cream (stored in the fridge) and stir until it's thoroughly combined. Next, slice the 3 large bananas and set aside.

Layer shortbread cookies and freshly sliced bananas in a glass dish. Pour half of the pudding mixture on top. Repeat this step with layering cookies, bananas, and pudding. Top with remaining whipped cream and garnish with shortbread crumbs. Refrigerate and enjoy!

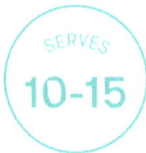

Classiq Tip:

Banana pudding is best served cold. I recommend keeping this cool for at least 5 hours before serving!

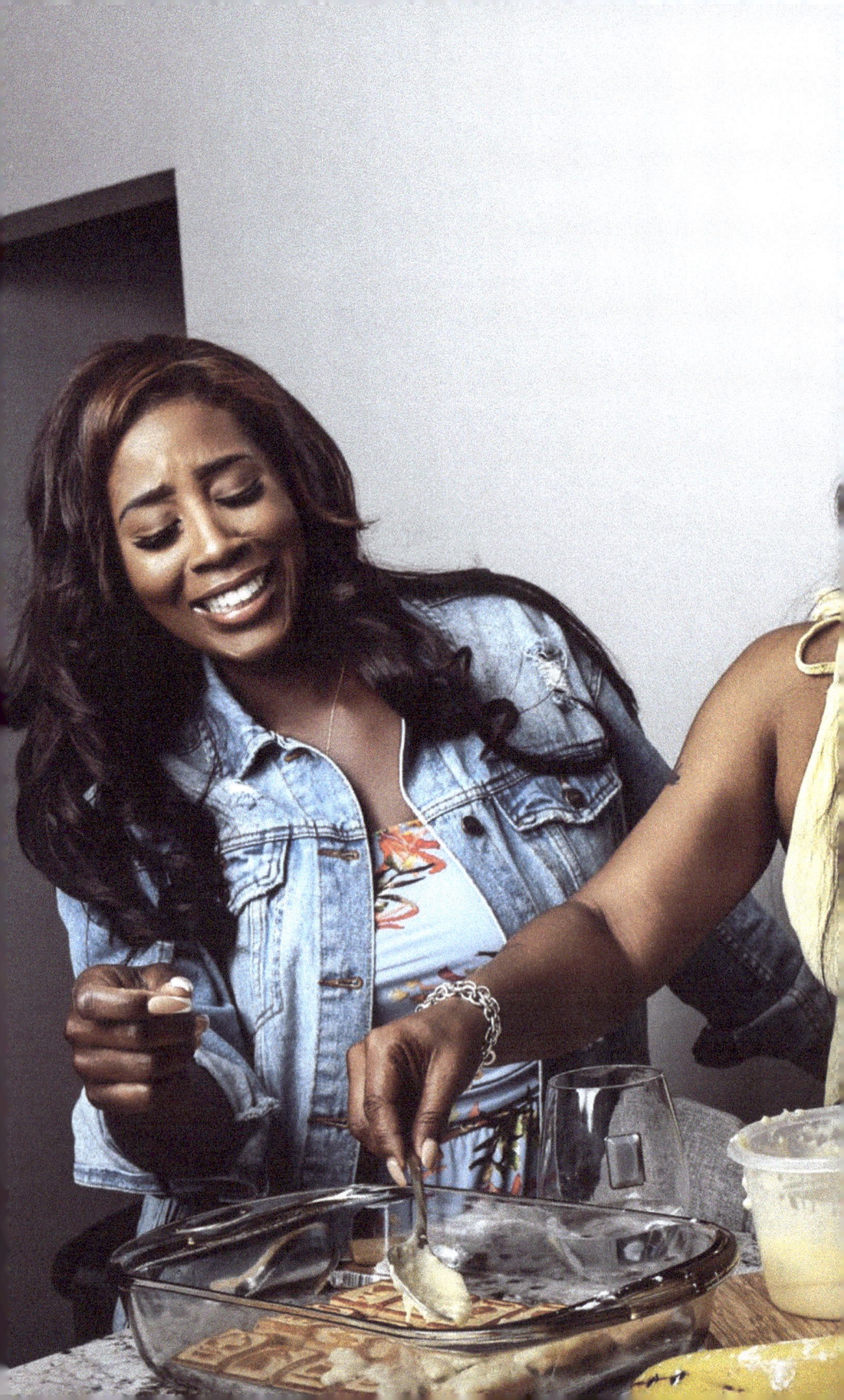

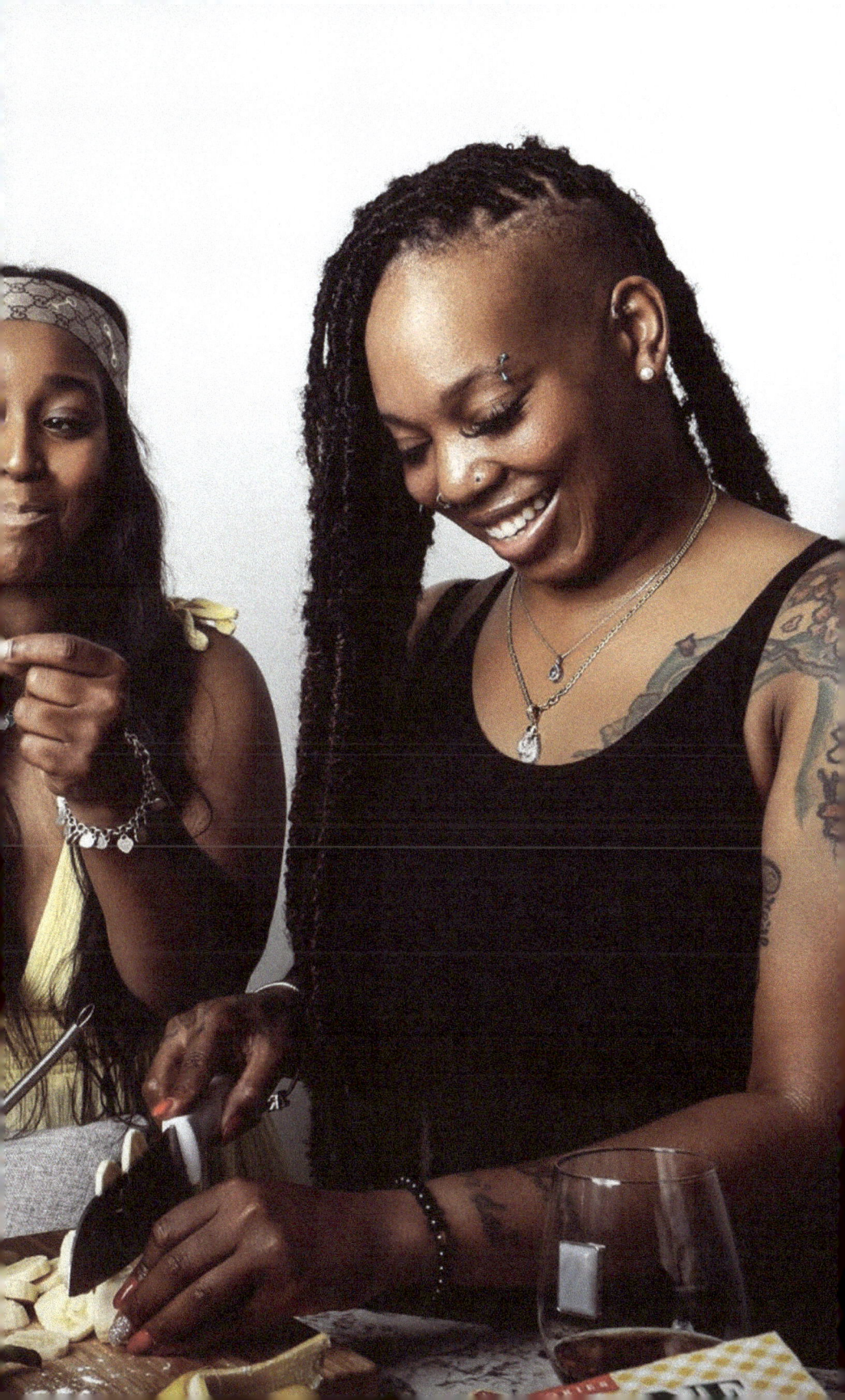

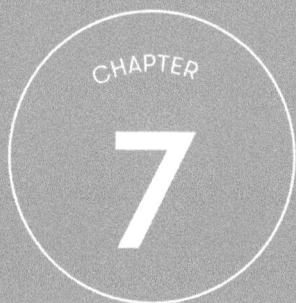

BONUS
RECIPES

JERK SEASONING

- 1 tbsp garlic powder
- 3 tsp cayenne pepper
- 2 tsp onion powder
- 2 tsp dried thyme
- 2 tsp dried parsley
- 2 tsp brown sugar
- 2 tsp salt
- ½ tsp black pepper
- 1 tsp paprika
- 1 tsp Accent
- ½ tsp dried crushed red pepper
- ½ tsp dried ground nutmeg
- ¼ tsp ground cinnamon

Whisk together all ingredients in a large mixing bowl and store for future use. The best way to store the seasoning is sealed tight in a zip lock bag. Or mason jar.

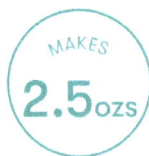

MAKES
2.5 OZS

Classiq Tip:

Jerk Seasoning has such prominent and lasting flavors that it's best when used as a dry rub. Use this for sweet, spicy and smokey recipes.

HONEY GLAZED SAUCE

- ¼ cup brown sugar
- 3 tbsp honey
- 2 tbsp soy sauce
- 2 tsp red crushed pepper
- 2 tbsp lemon juice

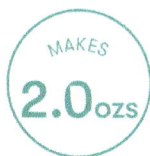

MAKES
2.0ozs

Whisk together brown sugar, honey, soy sauce, lemon juice and red crushed peppers in a small bowl until all the contents are blended.

"

Fruits & veggies are
the new soul food.

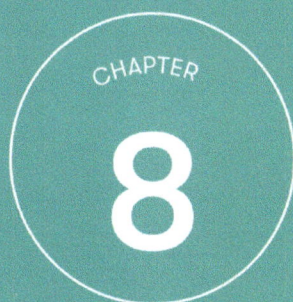

SMOOTH DRINKS

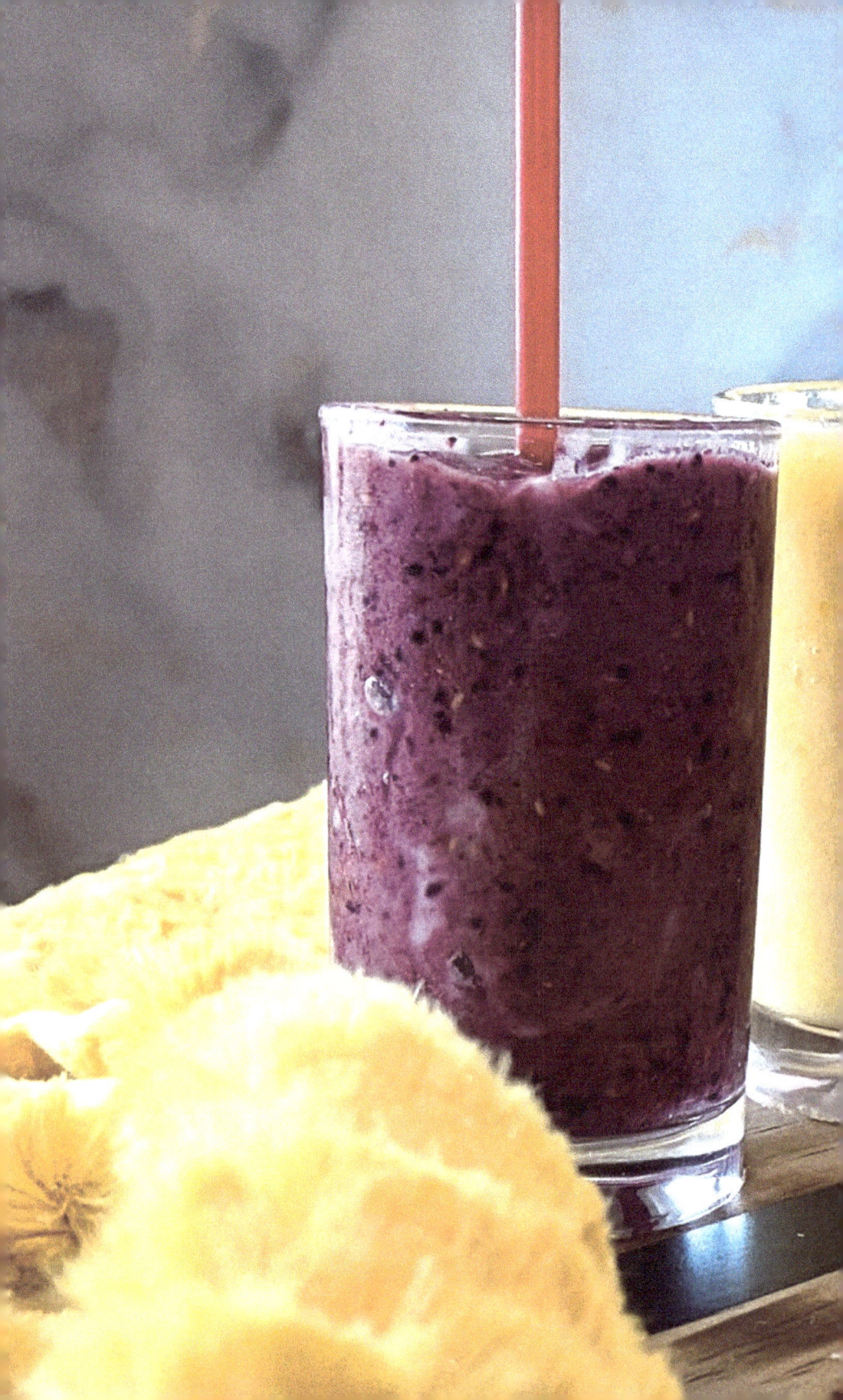

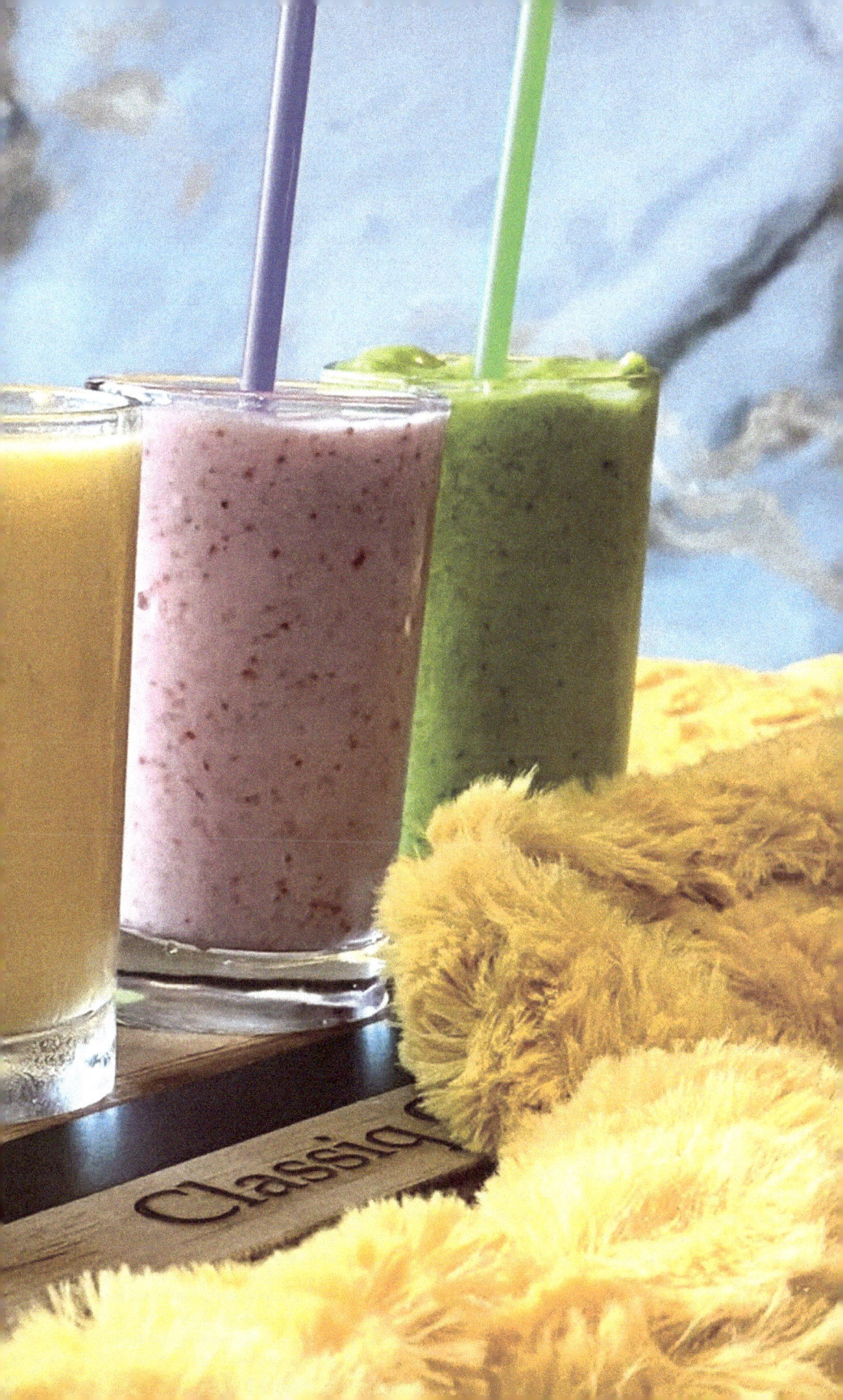

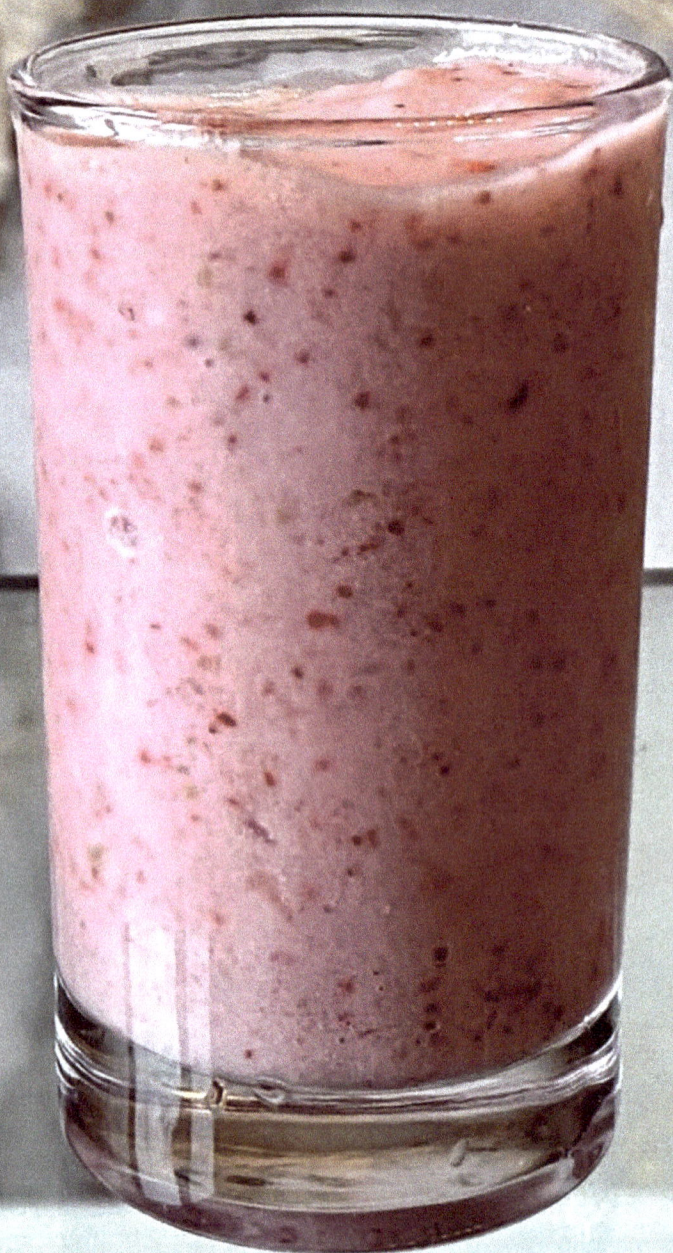

STRAWBAN
(Strawberry Banana)

- ½ cup frozen strawberries
- 1 whole banana (chunks)
- ½ cup strawberry yogurt
- ¾ cup almond milk

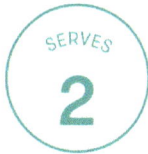

Throw yogurt into your blender and all fruit to follow. Top it off with your milk. Blend on high for 2-5 minutes or until you have a thick consistency.

SERVES
2

Classiq Tip:

For a looser consistency, blend for 5-8 minutes.

ALL BERRY GOOD
(Strawberry, Raspberry, Blackberry)

- ½ cup frozen strawberries
- ½ cup frozen raspberries
- ½ cup frozen blackberries
- ½ cup strawberry yogurt
- 1 cup almond milk
- 2 tbsp honey

Throw yogurt into your blender and all fruit to follow. Top it off with your milk and honey. Blend on high for 2-5 minutes or until you have a thick consistency.

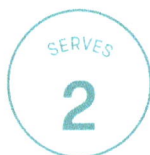

SERVES
2

Classiq Tip:

Fresh fruit is great to freeze and store for any future smoothies. It eliminates the need to use ice so that you can taste all natural flavors.

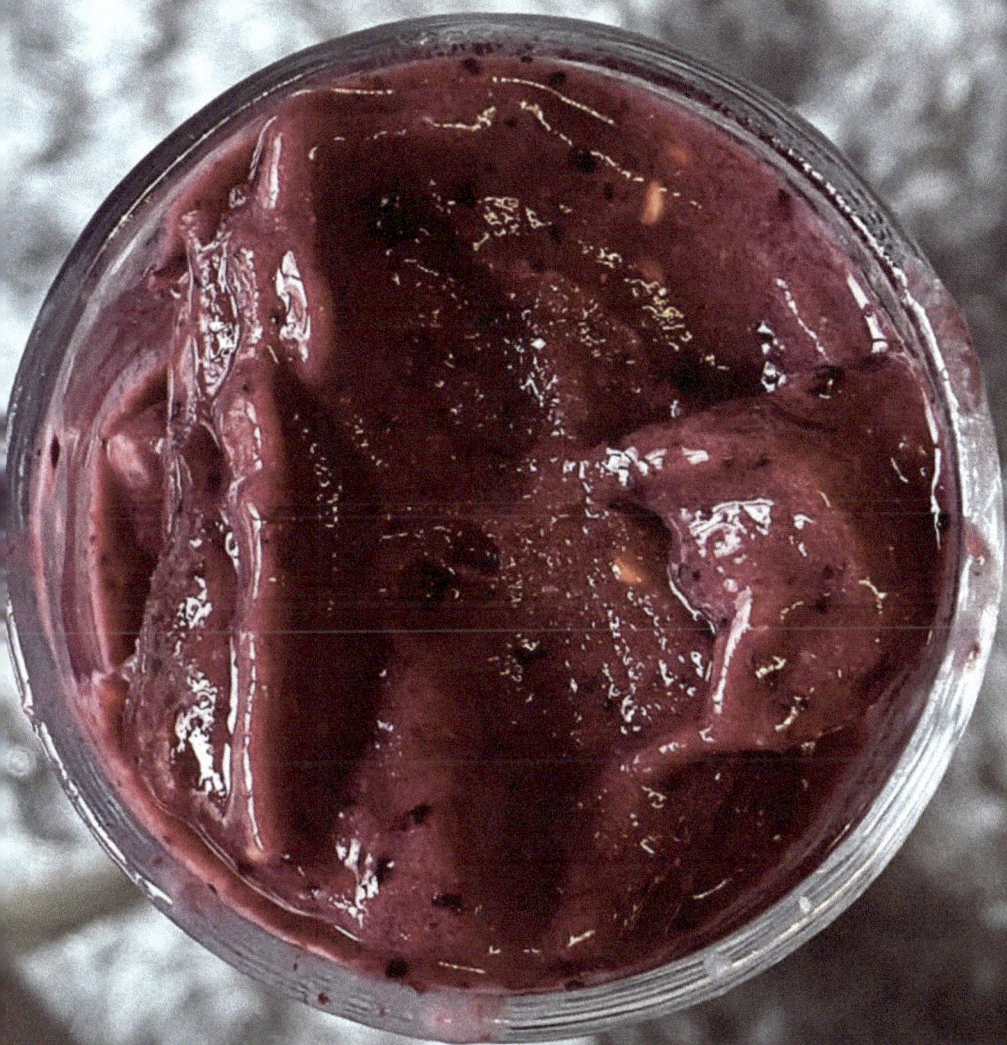

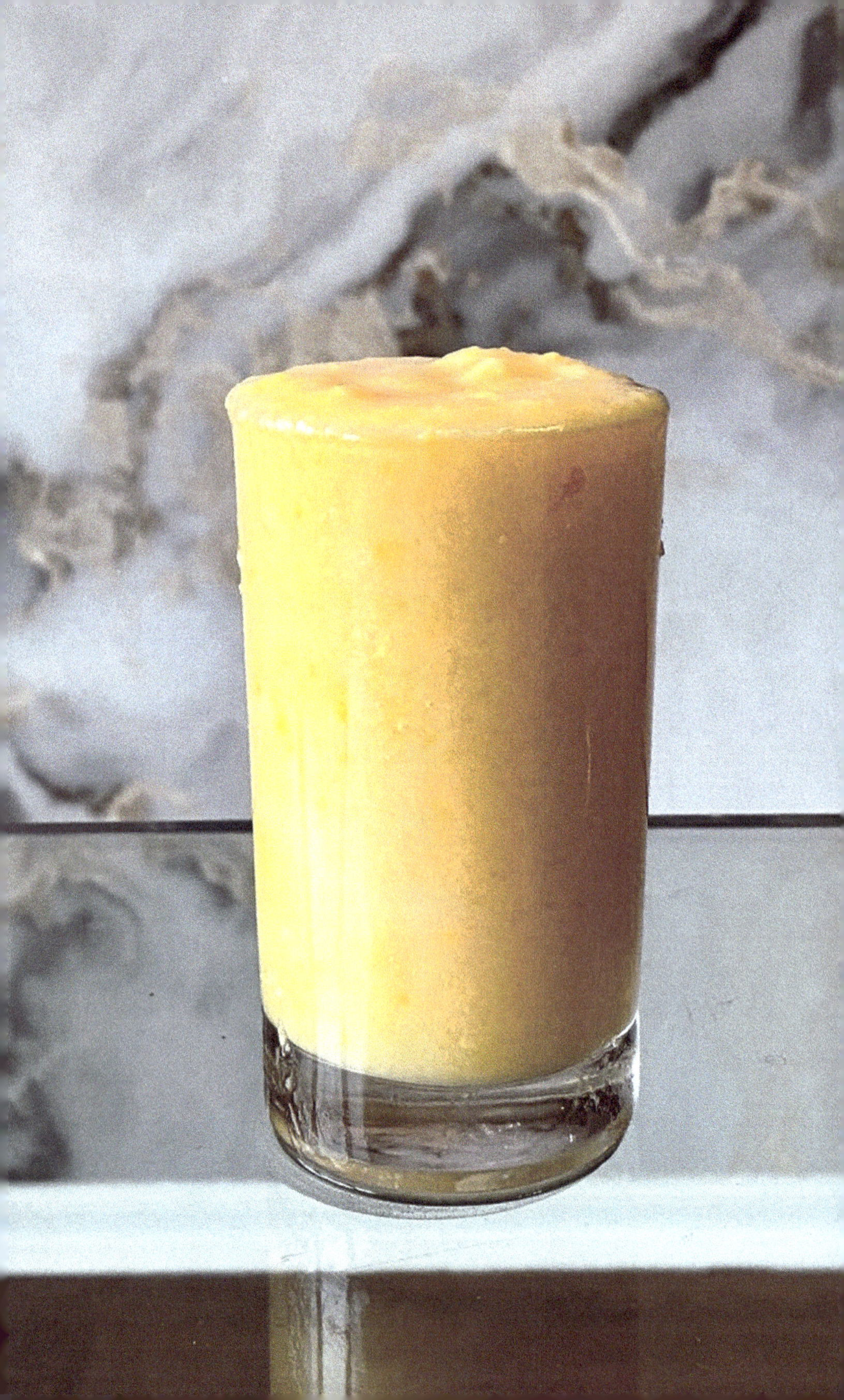

PMP
(Pineapple, Mango, Peach)

- ½ cup pineapple chunks
- ½ cup frozen mango slices
- ½ cup peach yogurt
- ¾ cup almond milk

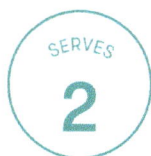

SERVES
2

Throw yogurt into your blender and all fruit to follow. Top it off with your milk. Blend on high for 2-5 minutes or until you have a thick consistency.

Classiq Tip:

The PMP is a great post workout drink. It's filling and is great to use as a meal replacement.

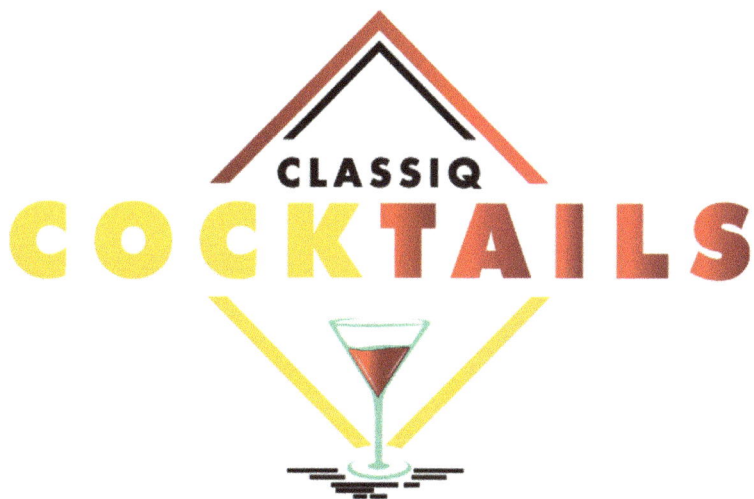

CLASSIQ
COCKTAILS

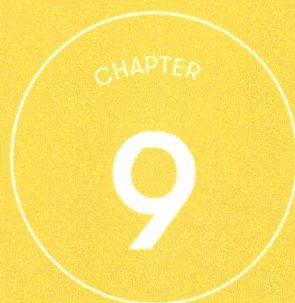

CLASSIQ COCKTAILS

» All cocktails can be turned into mocktails, just omit the alcohol or substitute for a sparkling alternative.

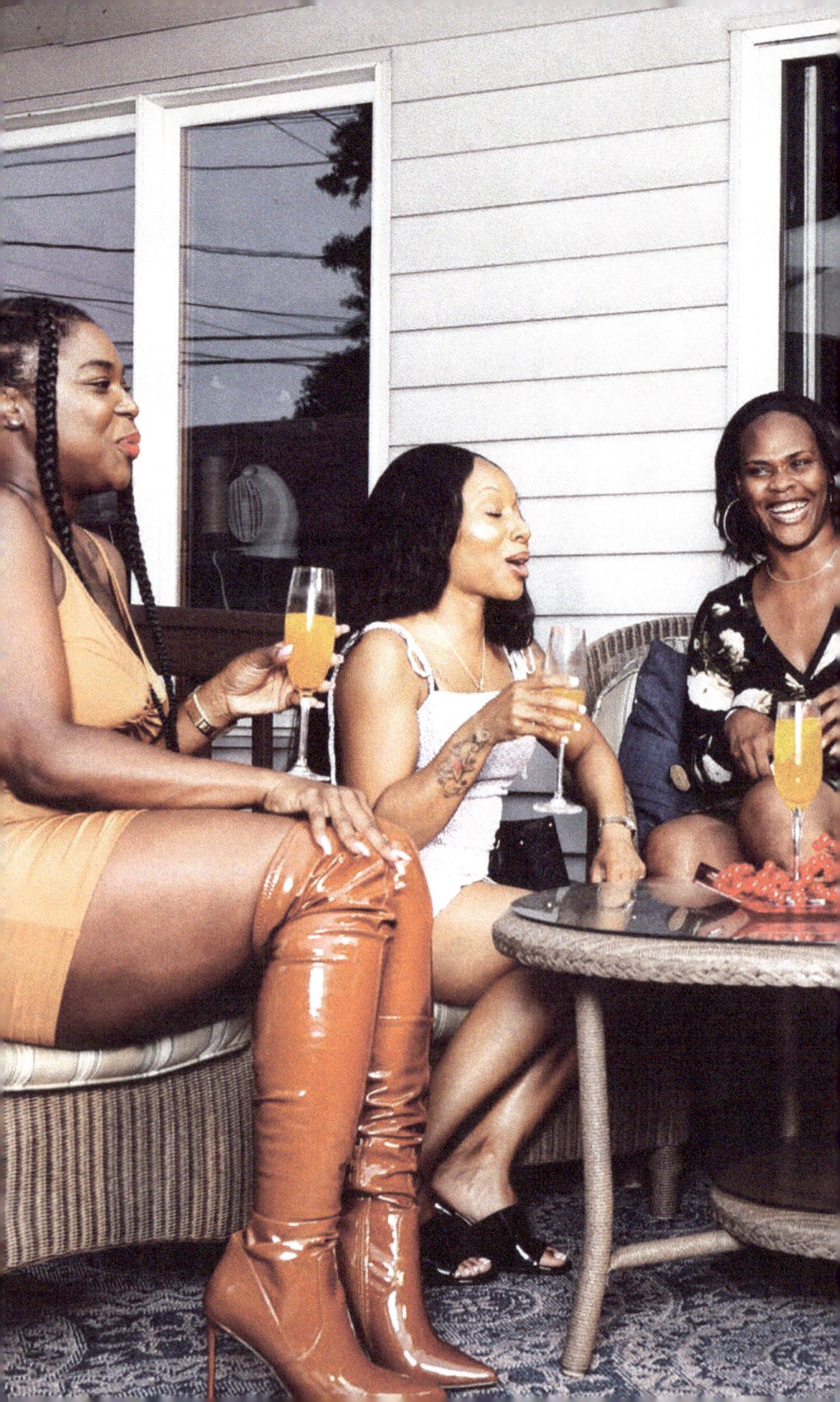

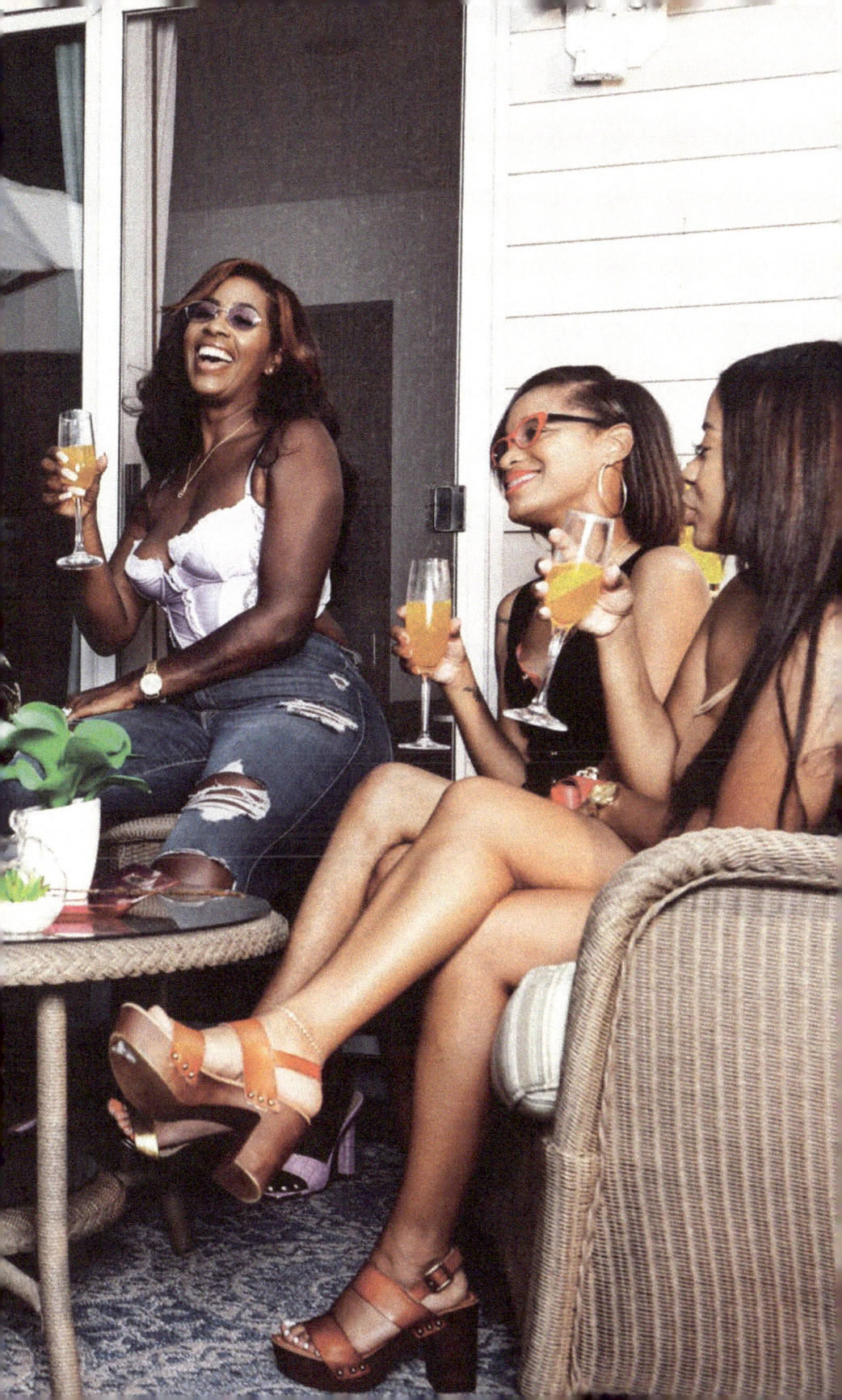

EM'S HENN

Honey, this is my go to drink. It's easy to make and tastes twice as good. Pair this with the Peppered "steak" over rice and you'll be thanking me later!

- Ice
- 1 shot Hennessy
- 3 ½ shots Tropicana's Pineapple Mango
- 2 tbsp lemon zest
- 2 tbsp cinnamon sugar
- 2 oranges slices

1 Shot = 1 Shot Glass

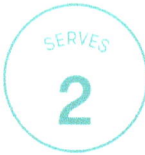

SERVES

2

Fill a shaker with ice. Pour Hennessy over ice and top with pineapple mango juice and shake well.

Fill a saucer with cinnamon sugar and lemon zest and mix well. Then take a martini glass and wet the rim. Hold the glass to about a 45 degree angle and slowly turn the glass in the sugar zest so that the outer edge is covered. Shake off all excess sugar and fill the glass with the drink mixture. Garnish with the orange slice and enjoy!

So how does it taste?

This drink has a sweet and fruity flavor. It's surprisingly simple to make.

MIRRITTA

Who's ready for a Mirritta? Please, make it two! This is the perfect summertime drink. Kick your feet up on the deck, feel the breeze run through your toes, and then take a sip of this and you'll think you're on vacation.

- Ice
- 1 shot Patron
- 1 ½ Daily's Cocktail margarita mix
- 2 tbsp sugar
- 2 lemon slices

1 Shot = 1 Shot Glass

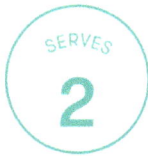

SERVES
2

Fill a shaker with ice. Pour Patron over ice and top with Daily's Cocktail Margarita mix and shake well.

Fill a saucer with sugar. Then take a margarita glass and wet the rim by squeezing a lemon slice around the rim. Next, hold the glass to about a 45 degree angle and slowly turn the glass in the sugar so that the outer edge is covered. Shake off all excess sugar and fill the glass with the drink mixture. Garnish with the lemon slice to the rim and enjoy!

So how does it taste?

Slightly sour, slightly sweet, 100% good!

CHERISHED PEARLS

For my peeps who like their drinks with a kick, this is the one for you! This drink is better than chocolate and guess what? All you need is one!

- Ice
- 1 shot Hennessy
- 1 shot Sweet Reggae Red wine
- 1 shot Triple Sec
- 2 lemon slices
- 2 Cherries

Fill a shaker with ice. Pour the Hennessy and red wine over the ice and top with triple sec. Shake well!

Fill the rocks glass with the drink mixture and garnish with a cherry and lemon slice to the rim. Enjoy!

1 Shot = 1 Shot Glass

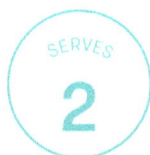

SERVES

2

So how does it taste?

This drink tastes like a perfect mixture of powerful and sweet. I usually make this before going out with my girls and dancing the night away.

KAY'S PLACE

How refreshing! The yummy strawberry and peach juice pairs well with the Martell. The popsicle is a bonus garnish. You won't understand how addicting this is until you try it. So go on... I dare ya!

- Ice
- 1 shot Martell
- 3 shots Tropicana's Strawberry Peach
- 2 Cherry Coke Popsicles

1 Shot = 1 Shot Glass

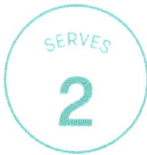

SERVES
2

Fill a shaker with ice. Pour the Martell and strawberry peach over the ice and shake well!

Fill the grange glass with the drink mixture and garnish with a cherry coke popsicle. Enjoy!

So how does it taste?

Sweet and smooth! Rich in taste and will surely make you smile until the very last drop.

FREAKY MEEKY

Judging by the name of this drink, you should be excited to taste it. This clever taste is the perfect blend of fruit and alcohol. Don't be ashamed, have two!

- Ice
- 1 shot Peach Ciroc
- 3 ½ shots Tropicana's Strawberry Peach
- 2 tsp Grand Marnier
- 2 tsp lemon juice
- 2 peach slices
- 2 mango slices

Fill a shaker with ice. Pour the Peach Ciroc, Grand Marnier, lemon juice and strawberry peach over the ice. Shake well!

Fill the martini glass with ice and pour in the drink mixture. Garnish with a peach and mango slice to the rim and enjoy!

1 Shot = 1 Shot Glass

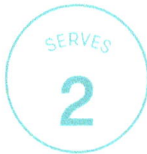

SERVES
2

So how does it taste?

It's the perfect winter drink. Its fruitful flavors and robust sweetness warms you up instantly.

MAMA'S PEACE

Add this drink to Sunday's brunch or at your next New Year's extravaganza. Whichever event you do decide to add it to, you won't regret it. The peaches and champagne pair well with ANY meal!

- 5 ozs Barefoot Bubbly Peach, chilled
- 2 ½ shots Simple Peach Bellini
- 2 peach slices (Ole Smoky Tennessee Moonshine is the brand I use)

Pour the Bubbly Peach in the flute glass and top with Bellini. Garnish with a peach slice to the rim and enjoy!

1 Shot = 1 Shot Glass

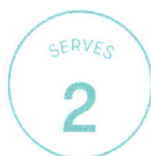

SERVES
2

So how does it taste?

Like Heaven! The light fizz adds the perfect kick to the flavorful peach. This is most definitely a fan favorite. Pair this with the Gourmet Breakfast Sandwich and you'll be spending less time at your favorite morning restaurant!

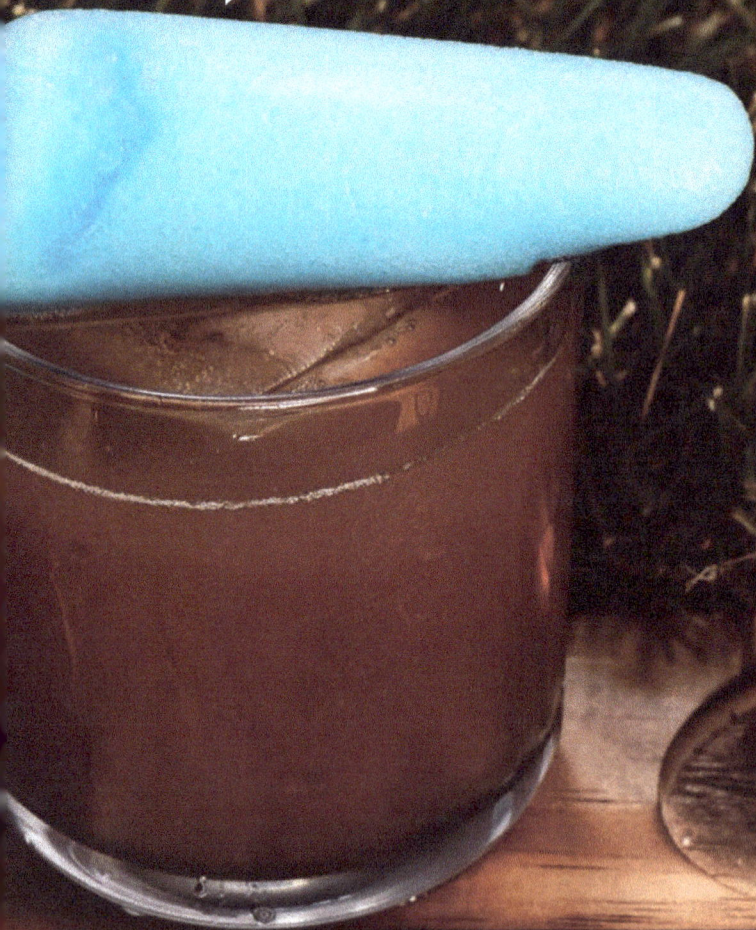
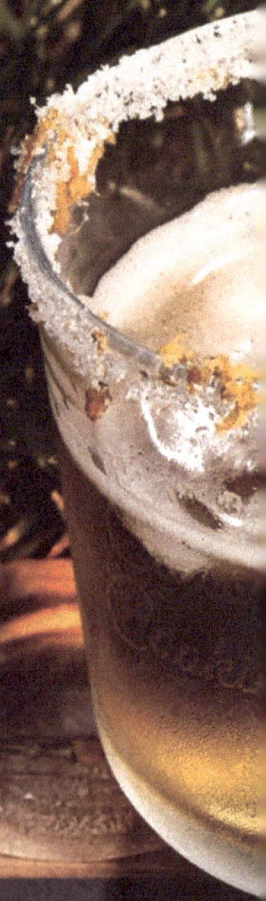
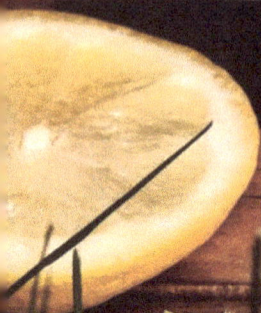

Classiq

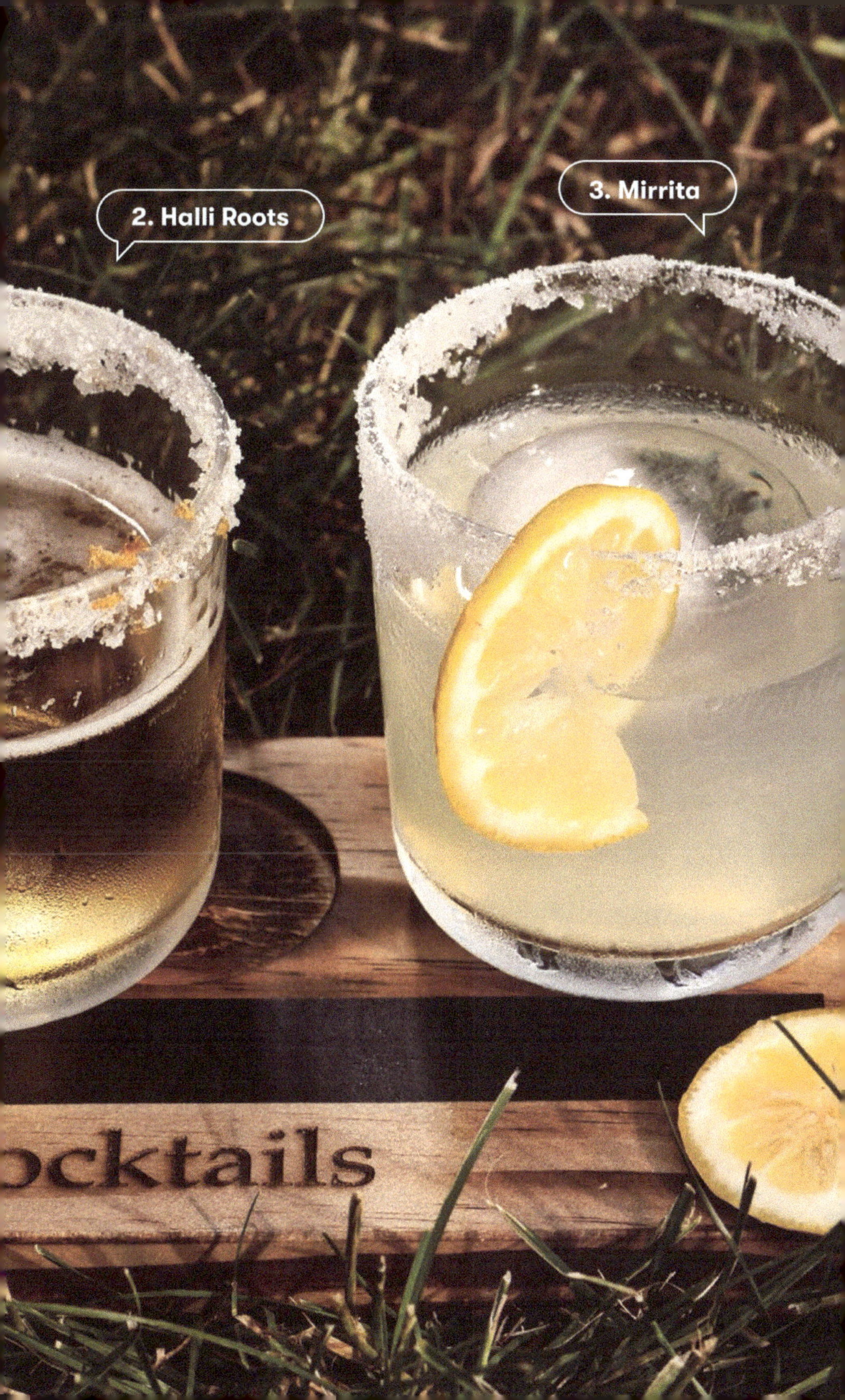
2. Halli Roots
3. Mirrita
ocktails

TY'S SON

This is such a vibe! Who would've thought that pineapples, mangos and Patron would pair so well? My tequila lovers love it and said they can't put it down. Tap in to this drink and tell me what you think.

- Ice
- 1 shot Patron
- 3 ½ shots Tropicana's Pineapple Mango
- 2 pineapple chunks
- 2 strawberry slices

1 Shot = 1 Shot Glass

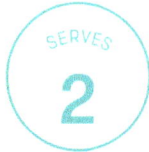

SERVES

2

Fill a shaker with ice and pour the Patron and pineapple mango over the ice. Shake well!

Fill the martini glass with the drink mixture and garnish with pineapple chunk and strawberry slice to the rim and enjoy!

So how does it taste?

A hint of lemon with a mixture of pineapples and mangos. It's the perfect tropical blend that we can't live without.

TOT'S T

Where Classiq meets unorthodox! You will literally crave this drink after you have your first sip. Every part of you wants to remain in control, but you won't be able to keep calm due to the rich and intense flavors. This is definitely one of my favs!

- Ice
- 1 shot D'usse
- 3 ½ shots Tropicana's Lively Lemonade
- 2 lemon slices
- 2 orange slices

1 Shot = 1 Shot Glass

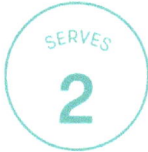

SERVES
2

Fill a shaker with ice. Pour D'usse over ice and top with lemonade. Shake well.

Fill a saucer with cinnamon sugar. Then take a balloon wine glass and wet the rim with the orange slice. Hold the glass to about a 45 degree angle and slowly turn the glass in the sugar so that the outer edge is covered. Shake off all excess cinnamon sugar and fill the glass with the drink mixture. Garnish with orange and lemon slices to the rim and enjoy!

So how does it taste?

This drink is sweet and tangy and reminds you of a sidecar. It's delicious and intoxicating!

HALLI ROOTS

Have you ever had a little party dancing in your mouth? Flavors that burst and explode with energy? This drink is extremely fun and will definitely impress a crowd!

- Ice
- 1 shot Jameson
- 2 ½ shots ginger ale
- 2 tbsp ginger root zest
- 2 tbsp sugar
- 2 mojito leaves

1 Shot = 1 Shot Glass

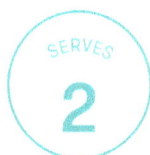

SERVES
2

Fill a shaker with ice. Pour Jameson over ice and top with ginger ale. Shake well.

Fill a saucer with ginger root zest and sugar and mix. Then take a grange glass and wet the rim with water. Hold the glass to about a 45 degree angle and slowly turn the glass in the sugar zest so that the outer edge is covered. Shake off all excess sugar and fill the glass with the drink mixture. Garnish with mojito leaf and sprinkle some of the ginger zest and sugar on top if desired. Enjoy!

So how does it taste?

Slightly bitter, slightly sweet and full of zest! Feature this drink at your next fire pit party and you'll have your guest addicted!

BRUNCH @ TIANA'S

This delightful drink has everything you want, plus more. It's the perfect blend of champagne and pineapple juice and will have you asking your favorite bartender to make Brunch @ Tiana's. Pinkies up for the classiq ones!

- **5 ozs Rossi champagne**
- **5 ozs pineapple juice, 100%**
- **1 tsp Rose's Grenadine**
- **1 pineapple slice**

Pour the champagne in the flute glass and top with pineapple juice and grenadine. Garnish with a pineapple slice to the rim and enjoy!

1 Shot = 1 Shot Glass

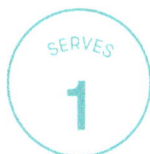

SERVES

1

So how does it taste?

Sharp, yet sweet. It's Classiq! Dive in and allow your tastebuds to take control.

THE NEWCOMB DROP

This drink reminds me of diamonds and pearls. Everything is rich in flavor and goes down ever so smoothly. By far one of the most refreshing drinks you'll EVER taste.

- Ice
- 1 shot Bacardi Limon
- 1 tsp Triple sec
- ½ shot lemon juice
- 3 tbsp sugar
- 2 tbsp lemon zest
- 2 lemon slices
- 2 quarter peppermints, crushed

1 Shot = 1 Shot Glass

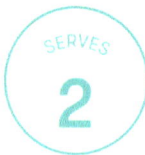

SERVES
2

Fill a shaker with ice. Pour Bacardi Limon, lemon juice and 1 tbsp of sugar over ice and top with Triple sec. Shake well!

Fill a saucer with lemon zest, sugar and crushed peppermints and mix well. Then take a martini glass and wet the rim using a lemon slice. Hold the glass to about a 45 degree angle and slowly turn the glass in the sugar and peppermint zest so that the outer edge is covered. Shake off all excess sugar and fill the glass with the drink mixture. Garnish with a lemon slice and enjoy!

So how does it taste?

Refreshing. Minty, sweet and sour. It's the best thing since sliced bread.

"

All happy endings
should include a
cocktail.

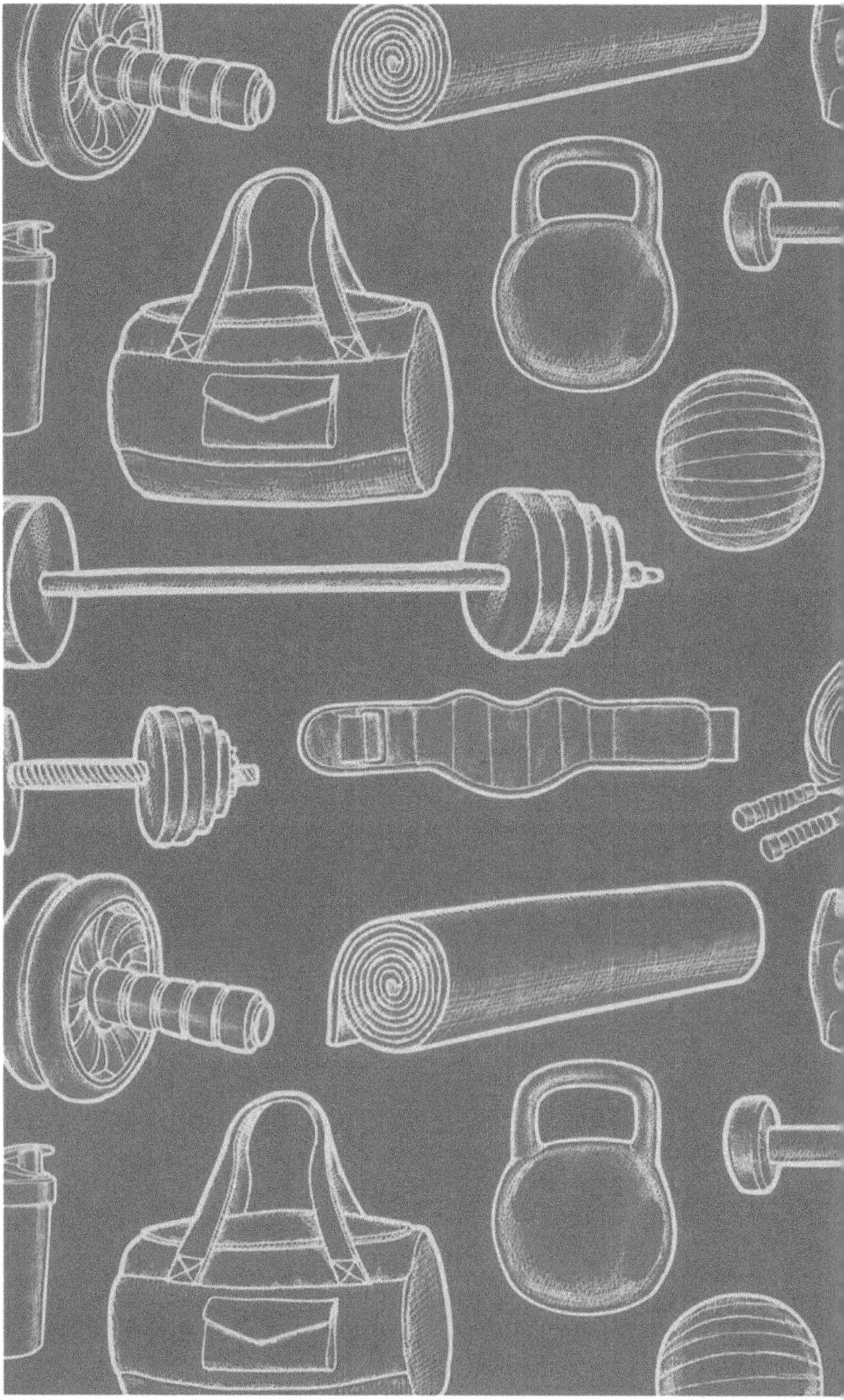

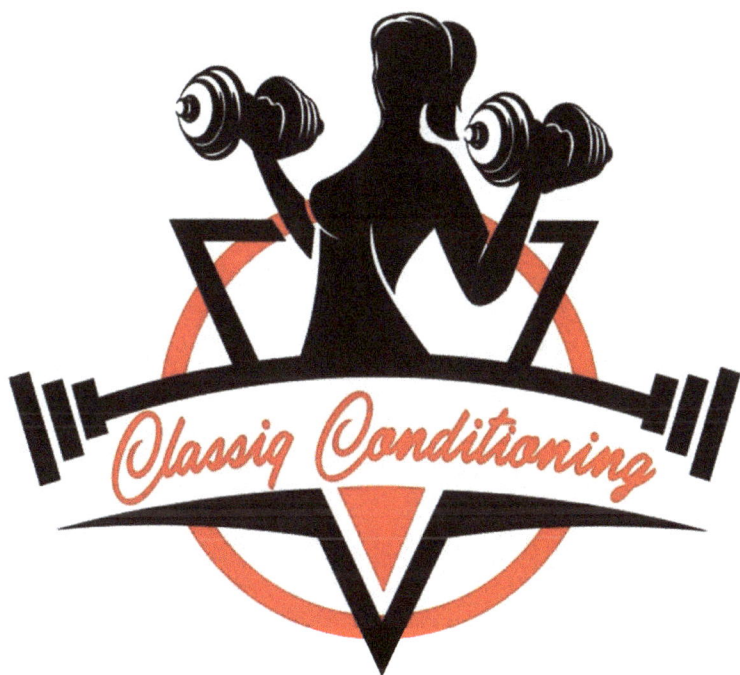

Although I love a good yet healthy meal, paired with a tasty drink, I honestly believe it's great to balance it all with a sound workout plan. I decided to include this portion because I know how much happiness fitness brings me and I hope I can encourage others to find love and enjoyment in fitness as well. It's important to incorporate fitness with a healthy diet because it helps lessen stress, increases your ability to focus, gives you energy and helps support your mental health amongst other beneficial factors.

CHAPTER

10

CLASSIQ
CONDITIONING

> ***Consult with your physician before embarking on any fitness routines, even the routines below***

Each workout level consists of 5 routines. You will repeat each routine for one minute and move on to the next routine. After you have completed all 5 routines, repeat the workout cycle for up to 3-5 rounds

LEVEL RANGES:

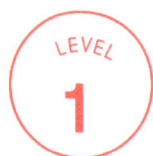 **Low**

I suggest starting at Level 1 for 3 rounds. Once you feel comfortable or need more of a challenge, bump it up to 5 rounds. When you have successfully completed Level 1 for a total of 5 rounds, move on to Level 2 starting with 3 rounds and so on.

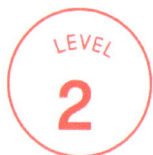 **Moderate**

To assist with aiding in a balanced lifestyle, try completing a 30-60 minute workout 3-5 times a week. Be sure to give yourself a recovery day in between. Try a nice walk, slight jog, stretching or simply resting will do.

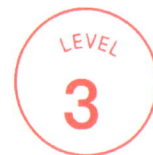 **Intense**

WORKOUT

» Jumping Jacks - 1:00 minute

» Sumo Squats (with dumb bells if available) - 1:00 minute

» Jump Rope (or high knees) - 1:00 minute

» Lateral pulls (with twisted towel) - 1:00 minute

» Walk out plank X shoulder taps - 1:00 minute

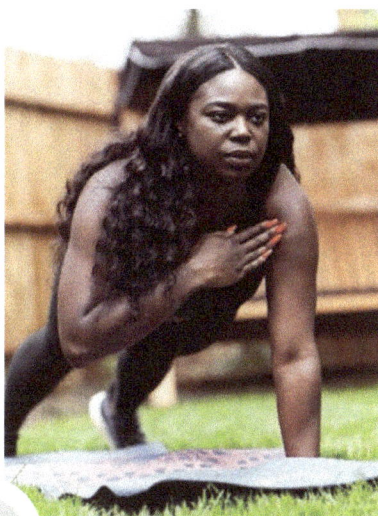

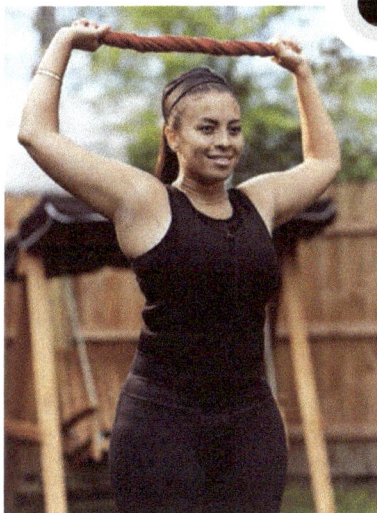

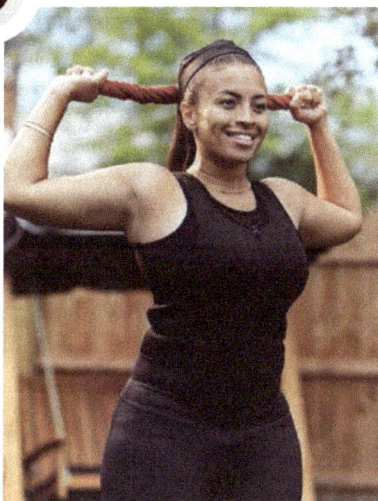

WORKOUT

LEVEL
2

» Seal Jacks - 1:00 minute

» Side Lunges - 1:00 minute

» Mountain Climbers - 1:00 minute

» Weighted Wall sits - 1:00 minute

» Burpee - 1:00 minute

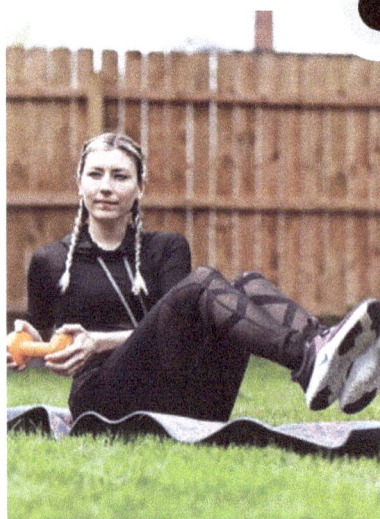
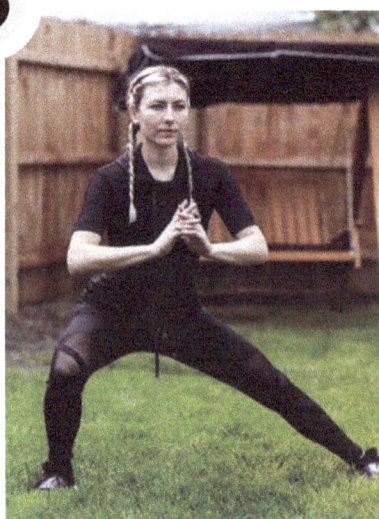

WORKOUT

LEVEL **3**

» High Jumps X Floor Touch - 1:00 minute

» Squat X Round Kick - 1:00 minute

» Russian Twist - 1:00 minute

» Fire Hydrant X Glute Kickback - 1:00 minute

» In and outs - 1:00 minute

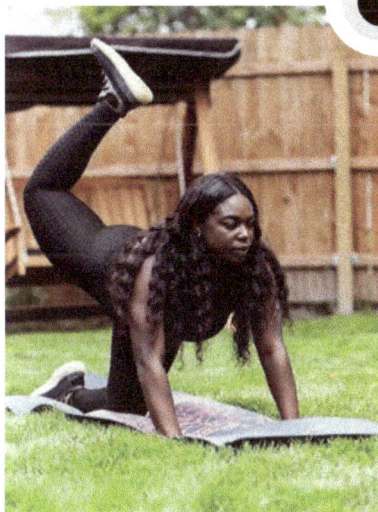
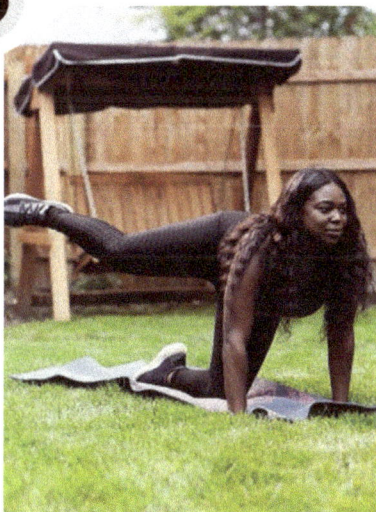

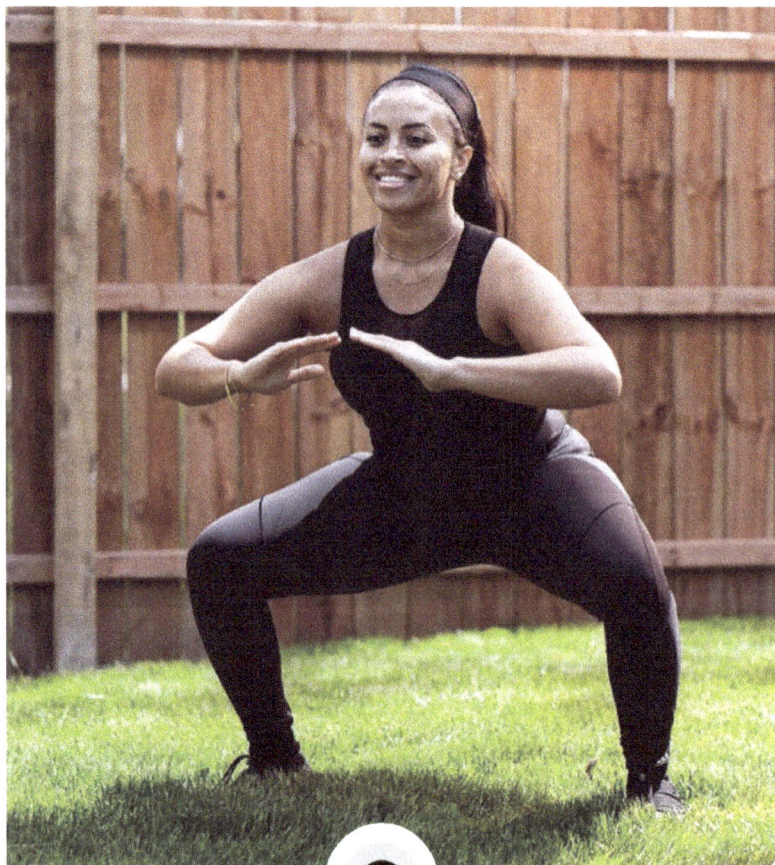

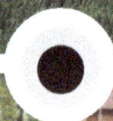

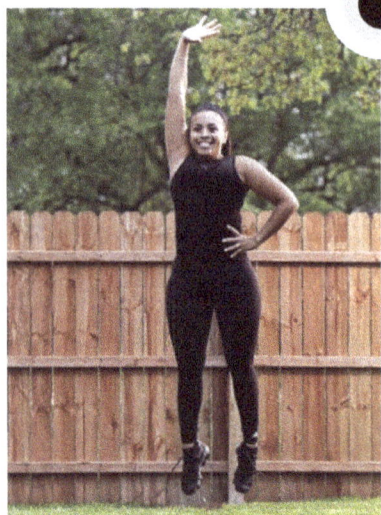

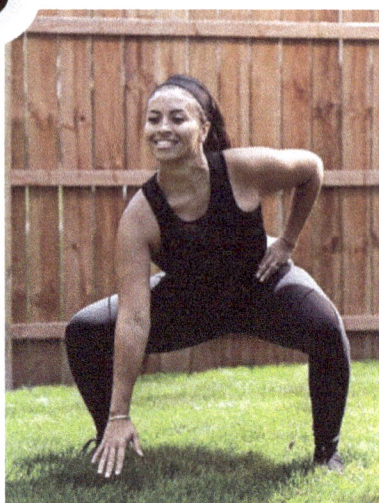

"

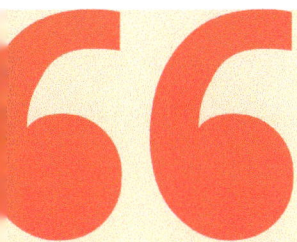

Don't stop! And when you feel like giving up, find that inner warrior and push through.

ABOUT THE AUTHOR

Native Clevelander, DawnDra Landon-Penn was raised by a single mother who worked three jobs to support her children. As a result, DawnDra spent countless hours in the kitchen, side by side with her beloved Grandma Bernice, while her mother worked. Surrounded by warmth, love, and encouragement, DawnDra learned to cook under the gentle and watchful guidance of her grandmother. She also drew inspiration from the other women in her family including her mother, aunties and siblings. Despite living in a neighborhood often described as a "food desert," there was always enough southern cooking on the table for the family. Classiq Cooking celebrates those cherished memories of family, love, and good times shared together at the table. When she is not cooking, DawnDra enjoys working out, concocting new drinks, singing, dancing and being a real estate agent.

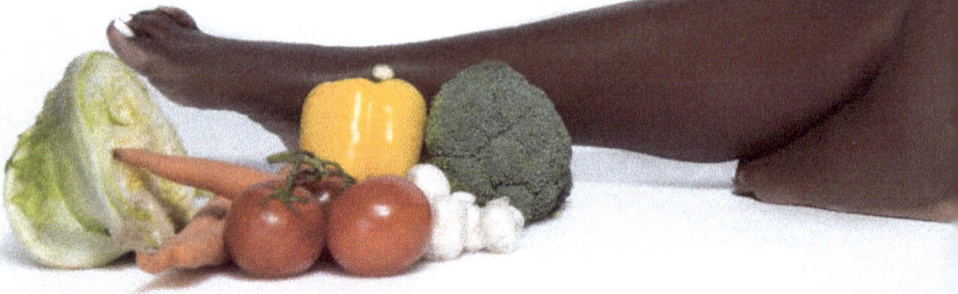

Visit her online at:
Dawn Classiq | www.dawnclassiq.com
dawnclassiq.booking@gmail.com

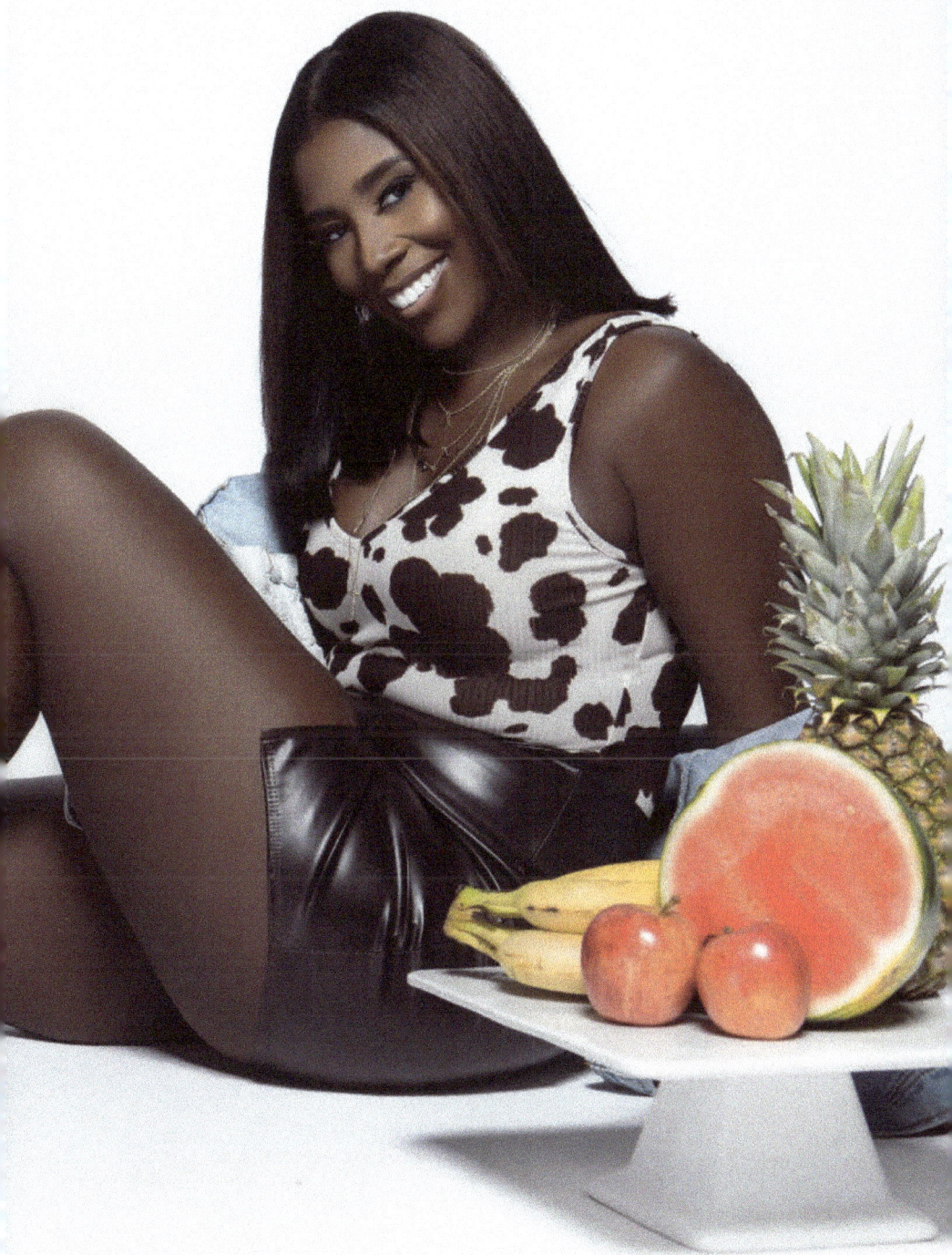

SPECIAL
THANKS

Agent - Raven Newcomb
Cover & Interior Designer - Daniel Ojedokun
Cover Photographer - Angelo Merendino
Editor - Mary N. Oluonye
Indexer - Zurain Shahzad
Interior Photographer - Anthony Davis
Interior Photographer - Michaela Penn

INDEX

S

U

Uncooked eggs
2
Uncooked white rice
54
Undercooked veggies
25
United States
66

V

Vanilla extract
5, 78
Vanilla pudding
78
Vegetable broth
38, 43, 56, 74
Veggie alfredo
51, 52
Veggie patty
3
Vitamins
13, 23

W

Walk out plank x shoulder taps
121
Walkers GF pure butter
shortbread brand
78

Watchful guidance
126
Weighted wall sits
122
White rice
38, 54, 60

Y

Yellow bell pepper
16, 24, 30, 43, 48, 60
Yummy Peanut Butter Bowl
15

Z

Zucchini noodles
48, 48

www.ingramcontent.com/pod-product-compliance
Lightning Source LLC
Chambersburg PA
CBHW041826090426

42811CB00010B/1123